300 Tips for Making Life with Multiple Sclerosis Easier

300 Tips for Making Life with Multiple Sclerosis Easier

Shelley Peterman Schwarz

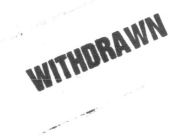

 Demos

Demos Medical Publishing, Inc., 386 Park Avenue South, New York, New York 10016

Library of Congress Cataloging-in-Publication Data

Schwarz, Shelley Peterman.
    300 tips for making life with multiple sclerosis easier / Shelley Peterman Schwarz.
        p. cm.
    ISBN 1-888799-23-4
    1. Multiple sclerosis—Popular works.   I. Title.   II. Title: Three hundred tips for making life with multiple sclerosis easier.
    RC377.S26   1999
    362.1'96834—dc21   99-17272
                                                                        CIP

Printed in Canada

DEDICATION

To Judy Ross, my mentor, cheerleader, and dear friend
Thank you for believing in me!

A special thanks to Tilney L. Marsh for her help editing this
book.

Contents

Foreword   xi

A Word from the Author   xiii

1. General Making Life Easier Tips   1

2. In Your Home   7

     I. Home Safety and Accessibility   8
         A. *Safety*   8
         B. *Lighting and Light Switches*   9
         C. *Doorknobs, Doors, and Doorways*   10
         D. *Under Lock and Key*   12
         E. *Ramps, Railings, Stairs, and Grab Bars*   12
         F. *Faucets and Sinks*   13
         G. *The Bathroom*   14
         H. *The Bedroom*   16
         I. *Furniture and Rugs*   18
         J. *Housecleaning Details*   18
         K. *Laundry*   19

II. Your Home Office—Computers and
    Technology   20

3. Looking Good, Feeling Better   **25**
    I. Grooming   26
    II. Dressing Tips   28
    III. Simple Clothing Alterations   30
    IV. Hose and Footwear   32
    V. Shopping for Clothes   34
        A. *General Clothes Shopping Tips*   34
        B. *Choosing the Right Clothing*   35
    VI. Accessories   37

4. Managing Mealtime Madness   **39**
    I. Making Your Kitchen More Accessible   40
    II. Meal Planning and Preparation   42
    III. Serving Meals   44
    IV. Streamlining Grocery Shopping   46
    V. Making and/or Using Simple Adaptive
        Devices at Mealtimes   48

5. Personal Empowerment   **51**
    I. Medical Issues   53
        A. *Record Keeping and Research*   53
        B. *Doctors' Appointments*   54
        C. *Medications and Medical Tests*   58
        D. *The Hospital*   62
        E. *Managing Your Home Health Care*   65
    II. Improving Memory and Cognition   67
    III. Quiet Restful Activities   72
        A. *Reading*   72
        B. *Watching Television*   73

C. *Playing Games*   74

IV. Weekend Getaways and Extended Travel 75

A. *Preparing for Your Trip*   75

B. *Traveling by Car*   77

C. *Air Travel*   79

D. *Foreign Travel*   82

E. *Packing*   82

F. *Staying at a Hotel or Motel*   83

G. *Out and About*   86

H. *Travel Resources*   87

6. **Additional Resources for People with Multiple Sclerosis**   **91**

About the Author   **103**

Index   **105**

Foreword

As the second millennium approaches (fondly known at Y2K), most people in this country are leading lives that are complex and frenetic. The imposition of a chronic condition such as multiple sclerosis (MS) may tip the delicate balance of daily activities into a situation that rapidly becomes unmanageable. The extra time needed to perform routine tasks not only is inconvenient but also may take the joy out of activities such as travel and recreation. Fatigue, perhaps the most common symptom encountered in MS, is also an impediment to getting things done efficiently.

In this book Shelley Peterman Schwarz shares with you 300 simple tips that will make your life easier. They grew out of her own experience of living with MS and its related disability, which gives them their "tried and true" flavor. Ideas span all aspects of daily life, from dressing and grooming to medical issues and recreation.

The happy result is time and energy saved, and frustration dramatically reduced. Shelley's tips will often surprise you with their simplicity and amaze you with their helpfulness.

Nancy Holland, Ed.D.
V.P. Clinical Programs,
National Multiple Sclerosis Society

A Word from the Author

Dear Reader,

On a dreary August day in 1979, I learned I had multiple sclerosis. I remember that day vividly. I remember what I wore, where I parked the car, how the drizzling rain helped hide the tears welling up in my eyes, and how my husband and I held each other after I told him.

At first I was relieved that there was a name for my minor but ever-present complaints: numbness and tingling up and down my spine, clumsy fingers, and an inability to run after the children as fast as I used to. Then reality hit and the fear took over. What about the future? How would MS change me and the life my husband and I shared? How would the illness affect our children, Jamie, age 5, and Andy, age 3?

A lot has happened since my diagnosis. The disease has left me with no use of my legs or dominant right arm. My weakened left hand can't even turn a doorknob or squeeze a tube of toothpaste. But despite all that, I'm happier now than I have ever been before and I live a remarkably unlimited life.

If you wonder how that is possible, let me try to explain. I think one of the reasons is that I've been a lifelong problem solver. Each time I face a problem, such as dressing myself independently, I take it as a personal challenge. Even today I look at obstacles and inabilities as problems waiting for a solution. After years of all sorts of personal and professional challenges, I have discovered that I am quite creative and resourceful. There are not many things I "can't" do.

This book is filled with tips, techniques, and shortcuts I learned from my own experience and from the people around me. Whether people were recovering from surgery, had chronic back problems, were pregnant, or just felt the effects of the aging process, everyone has his or her own ways of consolidating and streamlining simple everyday tasks. I became a keen observer of how other people did things.

About twelve years ago, I began writing down my personal tips and those I observed from other people. My nationally syndicated column, "Making Life Easier," is the result of years of problem solving. The column appears in newspapers and magazines around the country, including *Inside MS and Real Living with Multiple Sclerosis*.

When you live with a chronic illness like MS, it may be hard to predict good days and bad days, let alone the future. I hope these tips help you increase the number of good days you have and encourage you to develop your own techniques for making life easier. I am convinced that finding ways to adapt, modify, and simplify your life will give you the greatest opportunity to be happy and enjoy each day to the fullest.

Sincerely,
Shelley

P.S. I'd love to hear from you and learn how you're making life easier. Please send your tips to me c/o Shelley Peterman Schwarz, 9042 Aspen Grove Lane, Madison, WI 53717

(608) 274-4380 (phone)

(608) 274-6993 (fax)

<help@MakingLifeEasier.com>

<SPSchwarz@aol.com>

http://www.MakingLifeEasier.com

Chapter 1

General Tips for Making Life Easier

Being diagnosed with multiple sclerosis (MS) forced me to simplify my life. I was 32 years old and it was clear that life as I knew it had changed forever. As much as I wanted to deny it, I could not physically, mentally, or emotionally keep up the breakneck pace I demanded of myself.

As I began writing this book, I realized there were several overriding principles that everyone with a chronic medical condition like MS should know—for example, alternate periods of activity with periods of rest, plan ahead, and take advantage of labor-saving devices and new technology.

In this chapter you will learn the most basic lessons for conserving time and energy so you will have more time and energy for the things you *want* to do. Using these techniques, you will be more organized and be able to work smarter. And, most important, you will be more independent than you otherwise would have been.

☒ Keep balance in your life. Prioritize, eliminate, consolidate, and streamline activities in all aspects of your life.

☒ Take care of yourself. Make compromises. Do the things that are important to you and to your family and try to eliminate unnecessary or difficult tasks. Be sensible about how you spend your time and energy. Give yourself permission to rest. Put your feet up when possible and remove the word *should* from your vocabulary.

☒ Pace your activities and rest before you become exhausted. Try to break down a given activity into a series of smaller tasks or, if need be, enlist the help of others.

☒ Eat a healthy diet. Do not skip meals.

☒ Contact the National Multiple Sclerosis Society (NMSS) to find out about its client services and support groups. The NMSS can tell you about current research and treatments that will help you keep a positive attitude and give you hope for the future.

☒ Consider joining an MS or other support group. If going to an MS support group frightens you because you're afraid you will see others with more advanced cases and you don't think you can emotionally handle it, attend a newly diagnosed MS group. Or talk on the phone with people who have MS. Another alternative for getting the support you need is to contact a local hospital or clinic to see if they offer coping-type support groups for people with chronic illness or those who are going through life-altering changes.

☒ Use technology like cordless phones, speakerphones, answering machines, and wireless intercoms to save time and energy. For example, computers can be used for keeping records, keeping a journal, and writing letters. An Internet connection can expand your research capabilities from home and provide opportunities to communicate with others who have MS.

☒ Arrange your home for your convenience. Sometimes this means placing furniture in strategic locations to help you walk from room to room or placing a chair halfway down a long hallway so you can stop to rest. Sometimes it means purchasing duplicate cleaning supplies for the upstairs rooms and the downstairs rooms.

☒ When you need help, take advantage of products and services that are available. Don't look at this as giving in when you need something to help you. Instead, look at it as making intelligent decisions that will make your life easier and safer.

☒ Use labor-saving devices. Reachers, for example, come in various lengths, weights, and means of operation. Some have trigger grips similar to a pistol that are operated by squeezing your finger. Others have full-grasp handgrips that allow you to squeeze with all your fingers. I found one reacher with a locking mechanism that enables me to hold an object tightly without continuing to grasp the handle tightly. Some reachers have magnets at the end for picking up metal objects. Others have rubber grippers or vinyl-covered tips for better holding power. Battery-operated reachers automatically open and close gripping jaws with a light push on a rocker switch. Some reachers fold in half for traveling or storage, and some come with a carrying attachment that clamps the reacher to a walker or wheel-chair.

Many of the products I mention in this book are available in discount department stores, building supply stores, and home improvement stores. Unfortunately, many of the unique devices, such as tube pens to make writing easier or offset door hinges for making doorways wider, are not readily available in stores. However, there are ways you can locate these items.

Contact your local independent living center. Independent living centers are community-based organizations that assist people with disabilities to live independently. Every state has several. Your local NMSS office should be able to assist you in finding the center nearest you. Most centers have adaptive gadgets and devices you may borrow at no cost for a trial period. The centers also have a vast computer database of the companies and manufacturers that make these products.

Some NMSS chapters have loan closets for members to borrow devices to make daily living easier.

Call local medical supply companies, home health agencies, and/or hospital stores to see if they have devices in stock.

Contact a hospital rehabilitation department and speak with an occupational or physical therapist about the product for which you are looking.

Whenever possible, try out the device before purchasing it.

☒ When shopping, pushing a grocery cart may give you added stability as you walk. Some department stores have grocery carts for patrons to use, and a growing number of stores and shopping malls provide three-wheeled battery-operated scooters for shoppers who tire easily or have trouble walking. Scooters usually are available on a first-come, first-served basis at the service desk or information booth. Use the scooter to save energy.

☒ When noisy environments in restaurants, grocery stores, and department stores defeat you, select quieter places in which to spend your time. Look for places with drapes, low ceilings, and carpeted or vinyl floors. Avoid establishments that have wooden floors, loud background music, multiple TVs, or high unfinished ceilings. As a safeguard, carry earplugs in your purse or pocket.

☒ Before going out, call ahead to a restaurant, theater, new doctor's office, and so forth, and ask if the facility is handicap-accessible. Ask where the restrooms are located. Ask about parking facilities, about the most convenient entrance, and so on.

CHAPTER 2

In Your Home

I spend a great deal of time in my home, so I have tried to create an environment where I can be safe, independent, and productive. My home is now set up with widened doorways, ramps, lowered light switches, and touch-sensitive lamps. Although we have done two remodeling projects to add on to our house, the most valuable accessibility improvements have generally cost less than $50. Two of the simplest and least expensive are the following.

Shortly after my diagnosis, I found it easier to grasp and turn a doorknob if we wound several rubber bands around the largest part of the door-knob.

I learned that I could turn on and off all of my computer equipment—monitor, printer, and CPU—by pressing one switch if I plugged all of them into a six-outlet power strip. I put the power strip on the top of my desk within easy reach. You can put one within easy reach and use it to plug in a lamp, radio, TV, stereo, fan, and other items. You can find power strips with safety features such as circuit breakers or surge protectors at hardware stores and discount stores.

If your home needs some improvements to make it more accessible but you don't know where to start, ask your doctor to prescribe a professional evaluation by an occupational therapist (OT). The OT will come to your home and give you suggestions that will truly make a difference in how you use your time and energy to accomplish simple everyday tasks.

I. HOME SAFETY AND ACCESSIBILITY

A. Safety

☒ People who use power-dependent equipment such as oxygen, environment control units, electric beds and lifts, and so forth should notify their local utility company before an emergency power outage occurs. Your doctor will be asked to fill out a form indicating your medical problem and the type of equipment you use. In an emergency, the utility company will make every attempt to restore service as soon as possible. However, it still is your responsibility to have a backup power source. In addition, your local utility company will tag your meters so that when repairs, meter changes, or routine maintenance necessitate that the power be cut off, it will notify you ahead of time so you can make backup arrangements.

☒ It also is important to let your local fire department know if you might have difficulty escaping from your home in the event of a fire. If you have family members living with you, practice a fire drill at home. Show children how the smoke detector works and what it sounds like. Encourage your children to sleep with their doors closed because doing so will buy them time if there is a fire by keeping the smoke and heat out of the room. Be sure to discuss how important it might be to run to a neighbor's house to get help and call the fire department, emphasizing that leaving the house to get help would not mean they are abandoning their pets or family members. Contact your local fire department for more information on teaching home fire safety.

B. Lighting and Light Switches

☒ Replace traditional light switches with rocker-panel switches that require less fine motor control. They can be turned on or off by pressing with an arm, elbow, or palm of the hand, and are available lighted or unlighted. They are available at hardware and home-building supply stores.

☒ A dimmer switch allows you to adjust the light in a room so that one person may work or read without disturbing others.

☒ Wall switch extenders lower a light switch 13 to 15 inches below the actual switch, which makes it easy to turn on and off from a wheelchair. Some extenders mount over a standard single light switch, whereas others replace the existing wall plate using the same screws. The device is easy to attach and will not scratch or damage walls. A flat wooden spatula is good for extending your reach when you want to operate a light switch.

☒ Lamps are easier to turn on and off if you install a lamp converter, which bypasses the on-off switch and makes the lamp "touch-sensitive." The converter fits into the socket, and when you screw in a three-way light bulb, the lamp will light up when you touch it. With each successive touch the light gets brighter and then finally turns off.

C. Doorknobs, Doors, and Doorways

☒ Replace regular doorknobs with lever handles or purchase a rubber lever that fits over any standard doorknob. Lever handles are easy to operate—just push down with your hand, arm, or elbow. Or wrap several rubber bands around the largest part of the doorknob to increase its diameter. It will be easier to grasp.

☒ If the bathroom doorway is too narrow to accommodate a scooter or wheelchair, remove the door. Replace it with a tension rod and an opaque (or black) shower curtain for privacy. (This is an inexpensive solution to a temporary problem.)

☒ If you need to get around your home in a wheelchair, widen doorways by 1/2 inch to 3/4 inch by carefully prying off the door jamb strips on one or both sides of the door. Or you can install offset hinges to increase the door opening 2 to 3 inches, allowing the door to swing out and away from the doorway opening. To find out how to purchase offset hinges, contact a hospital's occupational therapy (OT) or physical therapy (PT) department. The hinges cost approximately $10.

☒ Keep door hinges well oiled. If a door scrapes along a rug, try planing it to make it open and close more easily. Another way to plane the bottom of a door is to put a large piece of sandpaper on the floor under the door (padding it with newspaper if necessary to create a good contact surface) and then move the door back and forth a few times.

☒ Make closing doors behind you easier using one of the following methods: (1) Tie some string or cord around the doorknob. Grab hold of it as you move through the doorway, and the door will shut behind you as you pull the string. (2) Attach one cup hook to the door near the knob and a second cup hook to the door jamb on the hinge side. Tie a string or chain between the hooks and pull it as you go through the doorway. The door will close behind you.

☒ Protect your doors from wheelchair scratches by installing a clear Lucite, chrome, or brass kick plate at their base. These are available wherever building supplies are sold or through home decorating catalogs.

D. Under Lock and Key

☒ Admit visitors without having to unlock or open your exterior door by keeping an extra garage door opener in the house. When you want to let someone in, press the garage door opener from inside the house and let your guest in through the garage entrance.

☒ Adaptive key devices fit on your regular key and give better leverage to make turning keys easier. Hardware stores and home healthcare stores have different styles from which to choose. Be sure to try them first to see which works best for you.

E. Ramps, Railings, Stairs, and Grab Bars

☒ Make your home easier to navigate by installing ramps, railings, and grab bars. If there is a door at the top or bottom of the ramp, there should be a level area in front of the door. A platform 5 feet wide by 3 feet long is recommended at the top of the ramp because it will enable a person in a wheelchair to unlock and open the door. Railing height above ramps is a matter of personal preference. The average-sized person usually finds that a height of 35 to 36 inches works well. If you are short, you may want to consider a railing 32 to 34 inches high. Railings should be on either side of the ramp. They should be 1 1/4 to 1 1/2 inches in diameter with 1 1/2 inch clearance from any obstruction, such as a wall.

☒ Before installing grab bars, determine where they would provide the most help. A space the width of a clenched fist should exist between the grab bar and the wall. Then be sure to anchor the grab bars to the studs in the wall so they can withstand the pressure and weight when being used. Vinyl-covered hand grab rails are better for grip and absorb less heat.

☒ Install hand railings on both sides of a stairway so you have support going up and down stairs. Basement stairs will be safer if you add abrasive rubber treads to each step. For added safety, paint the edge of the steps with luminous paint to make them more visible. To improve the lighting in the stair-well, use at least a 100-watt bulb.

☒ Save steps and attract the attention of someone who is in the basement by turning the light switch at the top of the stairs on and off a few times. The flashing lights will get the person's attention even if he or she has the volume on the TV or stereo cranked up.

F. Faucets and Sinks

☒ Turning water on and off is easier if you have a single lever arm to control the temperature and water pressure. Kitchen faucets generally have longer levers than bathroom models—and they are even easier to use.

☒ If you have separate controls for hot and cold water, consider installing wrist blades. Wrist blades are wide, wing-type handles that are operated by pushing with the forearm, wrist, or heel of the hand. They are available at most plumbing supply stores and hardware stores.

G. The Bathroom

☒ If you find the height of standard toilet seats to be a problem, purchase an adjustable portable toilet seat to increase the height 4 to 7 inches and make it easier to get on and off the toilet. They are easy to attach to any toilet. Some portable seats provide armrests for added support. Purchase a tote bag so you can take the seat with you and safely use bathrooms away from home.

☒ A wall-mounted toilet seat may be installed at a level that is convenient for you.

☒ Try these adaptations for safer, easier use of your shower and bathtub: (1) Consider a shower caddy, a hanging basket that hooks over the shower head and keeps soap and shampoo off the floor. (2) Use decorative nonslip tape or decals in the tub or shower for improved traction. (3) If you use a rubber mat, periodically toss it in the washing machine with soap and a little bleach to remove that slippery soap-film buildup. (4) Purchase one of the many inexpensive shower chairs available, or place an inexpensive resin or webbed outdoor chair in the tub or shower and have a seat while you bathe. (5) Never grab onto towel racks or soap dish holders for support. Install grab bars in the shower and bathtub. Grab bars must be securely anchored to wall studs. Get professional advice on the proper placement and hire a professional if you cannot do the installation yourself. (6) A metal hand-held shower nozzle may be slippery and hard to manage when your hands are soapy. You will have better control if you wind several rubber bands around the hand portion of the nozzle. (7) Shower curtains will slide more easily if you apply a coat of petroleum jelly to the rod and then rub off the excess with a paper towel.

☒ Improve your medicine chest and bathroom organization by doing any of the following: (1) Glue small magnets inside the medicine cabinet door to hold nail files, cuticle scissors, and other metal objects. (2) Use a spice rack placed at eye level to hold medications or small articles that might easily be lost in a closet. They will be easier to spot and you won't have to reach so far into the closet. (3) Turntables on the counter or in bathroom closets make items easy to retrieve. (4) Reserve a drawer in the bathroom for clean undergarments. That way, when you have finished showering, you have everything you need to start getting dressed.

☒ The medicine chest mirror may be too high for children or people who sit in a wheelchair. Purchase a telescoping mirror that either clamps to the side wall of the vanity or sits on top of the vanity counter. Telescoping mirrors feature adjustable, swivel-type necks that may easily be moved to various positions. One side has a regular mirror and the other side has a magnifying mirror, making it perfect for makeup application or shaving. Consider installing mirror tiles at various heights on the bathroom walls.

☒ Substitute a wash mitt or soft sponge for the usual washcloth. Sponges are easier to use if your hands are weak.

☒ Pop-up tissues are easier to grab than the kind that lie flat in the box.

☒ Keep a measuring spoon in one of the toothbrush holder slots for taking liquid medication. Or hang spoons from an adhesive-backed hook inside the medicine cabinet door.

H. The Bedroom

☒ To minimize the amount of walking involved, make one side of a bed completely, and then finish the other side. Use a 2-foot stick or a dowel with a cup hook attached to one end to help you arrange the blanket and sheet when you get in or out of bed. The hook allows you to arrange the bed coverings easily. However, you can't use the stick with an open-weave or thermal blanket because the hook snags the threads.

☒ You will be more comfortable in bed if you choose the right bedding and equipment for your needs. Always look for bed covers that provide warmth without weight. Woven knit sheets are easy to put on the mattress because the corners stretch easily, but if turning over in bed is difficult, woven satin sheets will help you slide more easily (especially if you wear nylon or silk pajamas).

☒ If turning over or changing sleeping positions in bed is difficult, consider pushing the side of the bed up against the bedroom wall and installing a railing or grab bar on the wall. Anchor the railing to a stud and install it at the height that makes turning easier.

☒ Keep a flashlight on your dresser by the entrance to your bedroom. Use it at night when you have turned off the light and need to illuminate the path to your bed. Then keep the flashlight on your nightstand so it will be handy if you need to get out of bed in the middle of the night.

☒ Organize bedroom closets for easy access by making top shelves and clothing rods low enough to reach without straining. Store items in transparent plastic containers to cut down on your search time. If you keep your shoes in shoeboxes, write a brief description of the shoe (e.g., "brown flats") in large letters on the cover to make locating the shoes easier.

I. Furniture and Rugs

☒ The best type of chair to sit on generally has an armrest, a firm shallow seat, and a relatively straight back. Use furniture that is sturdy and stable. Avoid low, overstuffed sofas and chairs because they are difficult to sit down in and stand up from. To make it easier to get up from a chair or sofa, furniture should be approximately 17 inches off the ground. Adjust the height of your furniture by removing casters or putting measured blocks of wood under each leg until the desired height is achieved. It is easier to get out of a chair by scooting forward to the edge of the seat, spreading your feet apart, and rocking back and forth to build up momentum.

☒ Remove throw rugs. Walking or wheeling on vinyl, ceramic, or wood floors is easier than walking or wheeling on thick carpet. However, vinyl, ceramic, or wood floors may be slippery when wet. If you install carpet, choose a flat, tightly woven, or tight loop style, not a plush, sculptured, or shag style, which make walking or wheeling difficult. Use a high density or commercial pad under the carpet.

J. Housecleaning Details

☒ Use adaptive equipment, such as extended handles for dusters or brushes, to sweep the kitchen floor while sitting. Or if you need to sit while sweeping the floor, use a child-sized broom. When dusting hard-to-reach places, attach a tube sock to a yardstick with rubber bands and enjoy the extended reach.

☒ Sweep kitchen floor crumbs into a pile, then wet a paper towel, wring it out, and use it to wipe up the crumbs. This technique works well if you can't coordinate the use of a dustpan and broom.

K. Laundry

☒ Have family members help with the laundry by posting an index card near the washer and dryer indicating how much and what kind of cleaning products to use, water levels, and temperature settings for each type of clothing. Remind them to keep Velcro™ fasteners closed so the garment does not collect lint or snag other garments.

☒ Collect clothes in one place and transfer them to the laundry area in a wheeled cart if possible.

☒ If the laundry area is in the basement, plan to remain there until the laundry is done, and have a place to relax while waiting. Hang clothes promptly after they dry to minimize the need for ironing. Sit down when you iron to save energy.

☒ When the laundry is dry, put it into individual laundry baskets labeled with each family member's name. Take the baskets into the family room and teach children how to fold their laundry and then put it away. Listen to music or a radio, or let children watch a favorite TV show as they fold.

II. YOUR HOME OFFICE—COMPUTERS AND TECHNOLOGY

☒ Have a routine. Get up and get dressed as if you were going out to work. Wear clothes that put you in an "I'm going to work" mood. Set work hours and keep to a schedule. If you want to work productively from home, keep the TV off. If you do not want to miss a particular program, set your video recorder and watch it at night.

☒ Create a work area where you can keep files, books, and other items you need when you work. Surround yourself with pictures, keepsakes, plants, music, and other pleasant things.

☒ Use small Lazy Susans on the desktop for pens, paper clips, tape rolls, staplers, and so forth.

☒ Computers offer several adaptive programs and devices to make using the computer possible for people with limited physical or sensory abilities, including (1) different types of keyboard configurations that allow you to type if you have a limited range of motion; (2) screen enlargers that enhance the picture from your computer monitor if your vision is limited; (3) screen reading software that reads aloud whatever text is displayed on the screen (for example, the newspaper, downloaded from the Internet); (4) word prediction software that helps you conserve energy by filling in a choice of commonly used words or phrases once you have typed in the first few letters of a word; (5) features like "Sticky Keys" on Microsoft's Windows® 95, which convert two simultaneous keystrokes into two separate, sequential keystrokes on the screen; and (6) voice-activated programs, such as Dragon Naturally Speaking™, which enable you to speak your thoughts directly onto the computer screen, dramatically reducing the time spent typing on a keyboard.

☒ Use a phone device that allows the receiver to rest on the shoulder and frees your hands during extended conversations, or use a headset that looks like a headband with a microphone and earphone. Use "big button" telephones with large buttons and raised or enlarged numbers and letters. Look for telephones with a volume control in the receiver. Some phones have "back-talk" devices that repeat the digits aloud after each key-press. Hands-free phones with built-in speakers and automatic dialing can be fitted with headsets and special on-off switches. You might find a cordless telephone with speakerphone, speed dialing, and intercom capabilities particularly helpful. Try using a speakerphone or preprogramming your tele-

phone to eliminate the need to dial frequently used numbers. Be sure to try out the
buttons of touch-tone phones before buying
one—some are easier to use than others. Also
consider the weight and shape of the
receiver because they vary greatly from
model to model.

☒ If you have trouble locating telephones with
these features, contact your local phone
company's special needs center.

☒ An extra-long telephone cord will let you
move the telephone to all parts of the room.
Eliminate hurried steps to answer the phone
by installing several telephone jack plugs so
you can always have a telephone within
easy reach, or let an answering machine
pick up the call. Also use the answering
machine to screen phone calls or to take
messages while you rest.

☒ You may be able to use your home telephone as an intercom. Here's how: dial your
telephone number, wait for the busy signal,
then hang up the receiver. All the phones in
your house will start ringing. When
someone in the house picks up the call, you
pick up the phone. The other person will be
on the extension. Today "revertive calling"
is available (free) in some areas of the
country. Call your local telephone company
and find out if and when this useful feature
will be available.

☒ Use a photo cube to keep the most frequently used telephone numbers handy. Jot
down the numbers and slide them into the
cube between the sponge and outside of the
cube. The cube is easy to locate and the
plastic keeps the numbers clean.

☒ Keep a magnifying glass near the telephone
as a handy aid when reading numbers from
the phone book. It will cut down on your
dialing mistakes.

☒ There are several things you can do to make
writing easier. (1) Take a rubber band and
twist it several times around a pencil. Roll
it into a position just below the area where
your fingers rest. The rubber band will help
you keep your grip. (2) Slip a 2-inch piece
of rubber tubing over the barrel of a pen or
pencil to make the grip easier to use. (3) Try
using pencil grips. Pencil grips are small
rectangular pieces of rubber with a hole in
the center. The pen fits through the hole
and you adjust the rubber grip until it is in
a comfortable writing position. It stays in
place until you move it or take it off. These
devices are found at office or school supply
stores. (4) Push a pen or pencil through a
practice golf ball to create a large grasping
surface. (5) Buy pens with a diameter of 1
1/2 inches (3 centimeters) because they are
easy to grasp and use.

CHAPTER 3

Looking Good, Feeling Better

The way I look and dress has always been important to me. After my MS diagnosis, however, I didn't have the strength or energy to shop and coordinate outfits like I used to. I wanted to continue to wear attractive, professional-looking clothing, so I found ways to adapt my old shopping techniques. One of the first things I did was have my colors analyzed by a professional color consultant. I knew some colors looked better on me than others, and I wanted to spend my limited energy looking for clothes that would be the most flattering. Once I knew what my best colors were, I carried color swatches with me when I shopped. An additional benefit was that eventually all the clothes in my closet went together and everything could be mixed and matched.

When I needed extra help, I began shopping at small clothing stores rather than large department stores because the sales clerks seemed to have more time to help me coordinate outfits and they also could help me in the fitting room. The clothing cost a bit more, but the special service was worth it.

On occasion, I have called a store to schedule a convenient time when a sales clerk could provide the personal service I needed. In some cities, stores offer personal shopping services. A personal shopper will listen to your clothing needs and specifications and find the appropriate items for you.

When Dave and I are invited to a special event or I just "need" something new in my closet, I no longer worry about shopping 'til I drop. I use a combination of store, catalog, Internet, and TV shopping and always find just what I want.

Use the following tips to help you streamline shopping, grooming, and dressing. When you look good, you will feel better.

I. GROOMING

☒ Bathing or showering in cool water is recommended for people with MS to keep body temperature down, but the idea is chilling! Start with warm or tepid water and gradually increase the coolness, giving your body time to adjust. Putting on a terry cloth bathrobe after showering is a shortcut to drying yourself, and it feels luxurious.

☒ Substitute lightweight cotton dishcloths for terry cloth washcloths. They are easier to wring out if your hands are weak.

☒ If possible, cut your toenails soon after you bathe because they will be less brittle and easier to cut. A toenail clipper or a pair of scissors with short blades works best. However, if your nails are too thick, select a heavy-duty pair or consider having them cut by a pedicurist or podiatrist.

☒ When bathing a child in a bathtub, kneel to reduce strain on your back. Always use your leg and arm muscles rather than your back muscles when lifting a child. If you are afraid to lift a wet, slippery child out of the tub, let the water out and dry the child off in the tub before lifting him or her out.

☒ Make combs, hairbrushes, and toothbrushes, easier to grasp by cementing bicycle-type handles to them. Handles are made of resilient vinyl and are good for either hand. Or build up handles with modeling clay.

☒ Dental floss "swords" look like the letter "C" at the end of a plastic toothpick, with floss stretched tight across the opening. They let you floss with one hand and are available in drugstores.

☒ After you buy a new bottle of nail polish, apply a bit of cold cream, vegetable oil, or petroleum jelly around the outside rim of the bottle. When you reopen the bottle, the top will come off easily and will not stick.

II. DRESSING TIPS

☒ Each night select and lay out your clothing for the next day. This will save you time and energy in the morning, and if you need help with buttons or zippers you will be able to ask a family member for assistance before he or she leaves for the day's activities.

☒ Choose what you wear based on the day's activities. If you plan on swimming, for example, choose an easy-on, easy-off outfit with few buttons, zippers, or ties. If you will be traveling by train or plane, wear an outfit made of a silky fabric. The slippery fabric makes it easier to move when you want to change your position. The same is true if you are traveling in a car with upholstered seats.

☒ Dress in front of a mirror. This will help you find the sleeves and match up buttons and buttonholes. Button garments from the bottom up so you are less likely to skip a button, or button the bottom buttons and put the garment on over your head.

☒ It will be easier to pull slacks up and down if you wear underwear made of nylon instead of cotton.

☒ Ladies, try wearing queen-sized pantyhose. The tummy portion is more generous than regular-sized pantyhose, which makes it easier to pull them up and down. (The leg

portion is sized normally.) You can eliminate wearing pantyhose altogether by
wearing knee-high stockings under slacks
and thigh-high stockings under dresses.
Both knee-high and thigh-high stockings
have elastic bands at the top.

☒ If you are inactive, you will be more likely to
feel cold. Dress in layers and you will have
better control over your body temperature.
The more loose-fitting layers, the better.
Spaces between layers trap warm air. Take
off or put on a layer as needed to keep yourself comfortable.

☒ Make a dressing stick by untwisting a wire
coat hanger with a pair of pliers. Use the
wire hook to pull on shirts and jackets.
Make your own zipper-pull by screwing a
small cup hook into a dowel.

☒ Always dress a disabled limb first. To
undress, take the garment off the good limb
first. Unbutton and ease the garment off
your shoulders. Reach behind your back and
gently tug the garment off.

☒ If you are wearing a cast, slip a section of
nylon stocking over the cast before dressing.

☒ To tie a necktie using only one hand, take a
bulldog clip or a spring-type clothespin and
use it to clip the narrow end of the necktie to
the front of your buttoned shirt. Then tie the
tie as usual. Once you have tied your

necktie, loosen it just enough so you can lift it over your head to put it on and take it off. To eliminate tying a necktie altogether, wear a clip-on tie.

☒ When dressing a child, have him or her stand on a footstool or sit on a countertop at a convenient height to reduce strain from bending and lifting. Buy children's clothing with front-opening zippers so children can more easily dress and undress themselves.

☒ Before you put on your socks in hot and/or humid weather, sprinkle talcum powder or baking soda in them.

☒ Put a plastic bag over your shoe before putting on your boots. The boots will slip on and off more easily and your feet will stay drier longer.

III. SIMPLE CLOTHING ALTERATIONS

☒ To keep long-sleeved shirts from bunching up at the elbows when you put on a jacket or sweater, sew loops inside the cuffs. Then grab onto a loop as you put your arm into the second garment. Tuck the loop up into the shirtsleeve when you're done. You also could try sewing loops of bias tape inside the waistband of slacks and trousers. Use the loops to pull pants up and down.

☒ Attach a small pendant, a locket, a key chain object, or a notebook ring to the zipper-pull on a jacket or sweater.

☒ Enlarge buttonholes and replace small buttons with larger buttons. Textured buttons are easier to manage than smooth ones.

☒ Use Velcro™ to replace buttons and other fasteners. Sew an existing buttonhole closed and sew the button on top of it. Then sew the soft fuzzy side of the Velcro™ on the underside of the closed-up buttonhole. Sew the other piece of Velcro™, the hard side with the small hooks, where the button used to be.

☒ Sew on buttons with elastic thread. (If buttoned cuff openings are too small to get your fist through, move the buttons to make the opening larger and/or sew the buttons on with elastic thread. The elastic thread will give the rebuttoned cuff opening an extra quarter inch or so.)

☒ Purchase or make a button hook by using a large safety pin. To button, hook one of the buttons with the closed safety pin. Then thread the safety pin through the buttonhole and the button will follow. You also may try opening up a metal paper clip and using one of the hooked ends to "catch" the button.

☒ Use Velcro™ or zippers to create openings in the side seams or inseams in slacks or trousers. They will be easier to put on and take off. To make skirts easier to put on and take off, open the back seam and sew in Velcro™ to keep the skirt seams together. The same technique may be possible on some dresses. Replace short zippers with long zippers to make openings larger.

IV. HOSE AND FOOTWEAR

☒ Support hose have a stronger compression (that is, they fit tighter to the leg) than regular hose. White elastic support stockings that hospital patients often wear have a stronger compression than support hose. Jobst™ stockings have the most compression. They require a doctor's prescription and special fitting.

☒ Wearing pantyhose with a cotton crotch eliminates the need to wear underpants in addition to your hose.

☒ Tube socks are easier to put on than socks that are shaped like a foot.

☒ Look for "footies" or slipper socks with nonskid tread on the bottom. Then you can walk on slippery floors without fear of falling. If you cannot find nonskid socks, use fabric paint—the kind that dries with puffy, raised lines—to create your own nonskid socks. Wear moon boots as slippers, especially if your feet always feel cold. Or look for fleece-lined or down-filled slippers.

☒ Sew loops into the inside of each sock and use them to pull on your socks.

☒ If you wear an ankle-foot brace that fits inside a shoe and goes up the calf, it will be easier to dress if you sew a 7-inch zipper into the inside side seam of your slacks.

☒ Shoemakers can change shoes that buckle or tie to Velcro™-closing shoes. They also can raise or lower heels and/or replace leather heels with rubber or crepe so shoes are not as slippery. If the tongue of the shoe keeps getting in the way, a shoemaker can stitch it to one side of the shoe or remove it altogether. Have the shoemaker sew a leather loop at the heel that you can grab to pull on your shoe. A shoemaker can enlarge the eyelets on shoes, which will make it easier to thread the laces. Or purchase elastic shoelaces. Consider having your children's tie-shoes converted to Velcro™-closing shoes if they are too young to tie their own shoes and your MS prevents you from doing it for them.

☒ Rub the soles of new leather shoes with sandpaper to reduce slipperiness. No sandpaper? Scrape the soles along concrete or stucco until the smooth sole surface is rough.

☒ If your feet are different sizes or if you wear an ankle-foot orthosis (AFO) on one foot, you will need to purchase mismated shoes. Ask your local shoe store if they carry them or if they can order them from nonretail companies like P.W. Miner (a drawback to P.W. Miner's special order shoes, however, is that they are nonreturnable). Also try the National Odd Shoe Exchange, which deals in donated shoes. Their address is 3200 N. Delaware, Chandler, AZ 85225-1100, (602) 841-6691.

IV. SHOPPING FOR CLOTHES

A. General Clothes Shopping Tips

☒ Out for a casual day at the mall and don't want to carry your jacket? Use the sleeves to tie the jacket around your waist. You won't get overheated and your hands will be free for other things. Or rent a locker. Lockers usually are located near the public restrooms.

☒ When entering an unfamiliar department store, immediately ask directions to save time and energy. Learn where the escalators, elevators, and restrooms are located.

☒ Find a fitting room with a chair and sit to try on clothes. If there is no chair, ask the salesperson to get one. If trying on clothes at a store is too difficult because of your energy level or physical disabilities, ask if you may take the clothes home "on approval" and try them on at your leisure.

☒ Instead of carrying your purchases around with you, have them mailed or delivered to your home. If going out to shop is not convenient, shop by mail. Visit the library and look through their many catalogs and mail-order brochures. Catalogs often contain measurement charts for your reference. Some bookstores have specialty catalogs for sale. Many companies have toll-free numbers for ordering merchandise.

B. Choosing the Right Clothing

☒ You will stay cooler if you wear white clothing when out in the sun. White reflects the sun's rays, whereas dark colors absorb them. Unfortunately, light-colored clothing is more likely to show soil and dirt, and that will mean doing more laundry.

☒ Clothing made of 100 percent cotton will shrink and need ironing to look fresh and crisp. Cotton blends with less than 50 percent cotton, on the other hand, need little or no ironing. Garments made of permanent press fabric require no ironing or special treatment. Read clothing labels before making your purchases.

☒ Knit fabrics are easier to get on and off than woven fabrics. In addition, knit fabrics are more comfortable to sit in and do not wrinkle as much as woven fabrics. Double-knit sweatpants with an elasticized waistband are particularly easy to wear and maintain. Purchase wool sweaters or jackets lined with a satiny fabric. If you have unlined slacks, purchase nylon pant liners to wear underneath. Some fabrics are actually "heavy," meaning they have weight. Clothing made of this type of fabric may tire you out just putting it on. Fabrics with a pile like velvet, corduroy, velour, and terry cloth make sliding on and off upholstered furniture more difficult. Nylon, rayon, satin, acetates, silk, and polished cotton make sliding easier.

☒ If you sit a great deal, purchase garments one size larger than you normally wear. The clothing will be more comfortable to sit in and easier to put on and remove. Clothing that is too tight may actually make you feel tired. When you find a garment you like in a style and size that fits, purchase several in various colors. This will save you time and energy in the long run.

☒ To help determine whether a garment will fit without trying it on, do one of the following: (1) Take along a garment that fits you when you go shopping. Match the side seams and length by laying one item on top of another. (2) Take your measurements at home and record them on a piece of paper you take with you to the store. Ask the clerk to measure the garment you have selected to see if it will work with your measurements. (Take a tape measure along with you.)

☒ Another alternative is to shop where maternity clothes are sold. The garments are generously sized and also are fashionable. Some of the new styles feature elastic panels hidden by pockets or a simple drawstring waistband. Caftans and muumuus are loose-fitting garments that look fashionable and accommodate fluctuations in weight.

☒ Shop for shoes after you have been on your feet for a while. Feet tend to swell as the day progresses.

VI. ACCESSORIES

☒ Clip-on earrings or earrings on a wire that do not need a back are more practical than standard pierced earrings for people who have the use of only one hand.

☒ A shoulder bag worn across the body (i.e., over the head) keeps hands free and allows you to transfer the weight of your purse from your hands or shoulders to your trunk. Slinging a purse over your left shoulder puts the weight on your right hip. Slinging it over your right shoulder puts the weight on your left hip.

☒ Purchase a hat and scarf combination or a hooded scarf to wear in cold weather. The scarf portion will keep the neck warm, and when not in use it can hang securely around your neck, leaving your hands free for other things.

CHAPTER 4

Managing Mealtime Madness

The kitchen is the busiest room in our house. Ever since my diagnosis, preparing and cooking meals has been a family affair. The children began learning at an early age how to plan meals, use appliances, cut and mix foods, cook, and clean up. When my MS reared its ugly head, the children had to do a little more while I sat on the sidelines providing encouragement and input. I was patient and accepting as they learned, and it paid off. When they went off to college and lived in apartments, they gladly chose the chore of making dinner, leaving the cleanup to their roommates. (As a bonus Jamie and Andy could make the foods they liked.)

In those early years I worked at making the kitchen more efficient and well-organized. I began by getting rid of broken or rarely used pots, pans, dishes, utensils, and so forth. Then I rearranged the remaining items, putting things where *I* thought they should be stored. I placed items close

to where they were used. For example, I placed silverware near the kitchen table, cookware near the
stove, and cleaning supplies near the sink. I
placed frequently used items in the front of the
cabinets and drawers and put seldom used items
in the back. If I used measuring spoons, paring
knives, or spatulas in different parts of the
kitchen, I purchased duplicates and kept them
where they were used.

Now that the children are off on their own,
Dave and I continue to work in the kitchen
together. Visiting friends and relatives also take an
active part in meal preparation and cleanup. And I
can't tell you the number of times they have said,
"What a great idea! I'm going to do the same thing
in my kitchen."

See if you can use some of the following tips
to manage mealtime madness in your home.

I. MAKING YOUR KITCHEN MORE ACCESSIBLE

☒ Place frequently used appliances such as
toasters or blenders on a countertop instead
of storing them in a cabinet.

☒ Use electrical appliances rather than manual
ones whenever possible, including food
processors, mixers, blenders, and can
openers. To operate an electric can opener
with one hand, put a piece of Styrofoam™
under the can to hold the can in place. Use a
different size piece of Styrofoam™ with different can sizes.

☒ If you have limited strength and have trouble opening a refrigerator door because the seal is too tight, place electrical tape across the bottom gasket of the refrigerator door in one or two places. The door will be easier to open. The downside is that the tape will reduce the door contact and may affect the energy efficiency of the appliance.

☒ Have various working levels in the kitchen area to accommodate various tasks, and evaluate working heights for maintaining good posture and preventing fatigue. Sit whenever possible while preparing meals or washing dishes, and use a large stool with casters that roll to eliminate unnecessary walking.

☒ Use wheeled utility carts or trays to transport numerous and/or heavy items.

☒ Hang utensils on pegboards or under cabinets to provide easier accessibility. Replace old kitchen gadgets and utensils with modern gadgets that have large, cushioned handle grips.

☒ If storage cabinets are deep and hard to reach, use lazy Susans or sliding drawers to bring supplies and utensils within easy reach.

☒ Use cookware designed for oven-to-table use to eliminate extra serving pieces. Use paper towels, plastic wrap, and aluminum foil to minimize cleanup.

☒ Use a cutting board with nails to hold items in place as they are being cut.

II. MEAL PLANNING AND PREPARATION

☒ Gather items needed to prepare a meal, then sit while doing the actual food preparation.

☒ Select foods that require minimal preparation—dehydrated, frozen, canned, packaged mixes, and so forth.

☒ Prepare a double batch of a recipe and freeze half for later use.

☒ Use a microwave oven or crockpot to cut down on cooking and cleanup time.

☒ If you have trouble putting clear plastic wrap tightly around a container you want to put in the microwave, try putting the food in a cereal bowl and setting a saucer on top of the bowl.

☒ Slide heavy items along the countertop rather than lifting them.

☒ Use a damp dishcloth or a sticky substance such as Dycem™ to keep a pot or bowl in place while stirring. You can purchase Dycem™ at home health stores.

☒ To open a jar when your hands are weak, purchase a 5 inch × 5 inch thin waffle-like sheet where kitchen gadgets are sold. These rubberized sheets make untwisting caps and lids easier. In addition, put grippers under a floor mat or a throw rug to keep it in place. The sheets may be cut to fit any size or shape, and a package of four costs approximately $2. Another way to make opening jars easier is to put on a rubber glove before twisting. Or try winding a thick rubber band twice around the lid for improved grip.

☒ Line baking pans with foil to minimize cleanup, and soak pots and pans to eliminate scrubbing.

☒ Bake rather than fry whenever possible. Not only will the meal be healthier, but cooking it will be safer for you.

☒ Bake drop cookies as bar cookies. Spread all the cookie dough on a jelly-roll pan. Then bake and cut the baked cookies into squares.

☒ Prepare marinated meats, which are easier to cut and chew. If chewing is a problem, foods like carrots and other hard vegetables or tough meats may be chopped, steamed, stewed, ground, or grated to make them easier to chew without losing their nutritional value.

☒ Enlist help in the kitchen. When you involve your children in cooking and other mealtime preparations, remember that things that are obvious to adults may not always be obvious to children. For example, there is a vast difference between sugar and salt, but they both look like tiny white crystals, so children might substitute one for the other. Be sure to allow extra time when helping children learn to cook. There may be a mishap and you will need extra time to fix the mistake. Keep the atmosphere light and your sense of humor intact.

☒ Promote teamwork at mealtime and give everyone a job to do. At cleanup time the rule should be that no one leaves the kitchen until everyone leaves.

☒ There is some evidence that a low-fat diet is beneficial to people with MS. Try to limit your fat intake to 30 grams or less per day. Read labels and make simple changes in your diet such as having salad dressing served on the side, eating baked or steamed foods rather than fried foods, eating more fresh fruits and vegetables, and reducing your intake of processed foods.

III. SERVING MEALS

☒ Use Melamine™ or Corelle™ dishes whenever possible if you don't use paper plates. They are lighter weight and do not break as easily as china plates.

☒ Dishes and flatware that contrast with the color of the tabletop will be easier to find and will make eating easier.

☒ Use a dish towel or hand towel on your lap instead of a napkin. They are bigger and more absorbent, and are less likely to fall on the floor. For a quickie apron for an adult or child, fold a bath towel in half and put a string around it and tie it under the arms. It gives all-over double protection.

☒ Cutting pizza into squares makes it easier to handle and eat than traditional triangles.

☒ Eliminate your sugar bowl altogether. To avoid spills and waste, fill a large kitchen salt shaker with sugar. Be sure to label it. It's easier to handle and control the flow.

☒ Reduce stress at mealtime with children by giving them some choices. When serving new foods, ask if they want the "new stuff" in one mountain or two. Do they want the sandwiches cut in halves or in quarters? Do they want to try the vegetable now or before their bedtime snack?

☒ Use a muffin pan to hold condiments such as mustard, ketchup, relish, and onions so you won't have to pass around a lot of jars.

☒ To make cleanup easier for you and for your "little helpers," place a platform in the bottom of your sink basin if it is too deep to reach without straining. The platform can be made from strips of wood, or you could purchase a plastic tub or baking dish and invert it so that it raises the sink bottom by a few inches. If the tub or dish does not quite fit your sink dimensions, try placing a cooling rack that fits snugly to the sink over the tub so dishes won't fall to the sides.

☒ When unloading the dishwasher, set the table with the dishes and silverware you will need for the next meal.

IV. STREAMLINING GROCERY SHOPPING

☒ Plan menus for the week before going to the store, and take a shopping list with you. Write your list on an envelope, and keep coupons inside the envelope. Have two lists—one for high-priority items and the other for non-essentials or other items that might wait if you are suddenly overcome with fatigue while shopping.

☒ Choose a grocery store that will not defeat you before you begin. When deciding on a store, take into account not only prices and location but also layout and facilities, including restrooms. Is the store accessible?

☒ Use the same grocery store on a regular basis, and learn where various items are located for easier shopping. If you make a master grocery list organized to match the store's layout (indicating, for example, what products are in each aisle), you can save time and energy by photocopying the list and simply checking off the specific items you need. That way, the next time you or someone assisting you goes shopping, there will be no question as to which items you need and where they can be found.

☒ If you need assistance reaching items on a shelf, ask a nearby shopper or a salesperson for help. Some stores will have an employee accompany you as you shop. Contact the store manager or owner to arrange for any special services you might need.

☒ Take along a magnifying glass on a cord or chain around your neck. The small print on products can easily be read and compared with other brands.

☒ If an item at the meat or produce counter is too large, ask an employee to divide and repackage it into smaller, more manageable portions.

☒ Ask the bagger not to fill your bags too full. Spread out the items into more, but lighter-weight, bags. Ask that all frozen or perishable foods be put into one bag. Then when you arrive home you only need to empty one bag immediately, and the others can wait.

☒ Call a small grocery store with your order. Tell them when you will be there to pick it up, and if you can't leave your car, tell them that you will have your lights on or honk your horn when you arrive in the parking lot. Generally, small stores are able to make deliveries to your car if notified in advance.

You also may want to ask them what time of the day would be most convenient for you to drive over to pick up your order. Some stores offer home delivery, which is especially helpful if you cannot drive or the weather is too hot or cold to venture out. Check out Internet grocery services, too.

V MAKING AND/OR USING SIMPLE ADAPTIVE DEVICES AT MEALTIMES

☒ If grasping and holding onto silverware is difficult, use modeling clay to build up the handles. Or cement the handles in bicycle handle grips, which are shaped to accommodate the individual fingers. Purchase stainless steel flatware with big bamboo or plastic handles that are easier to grip.

☒ Use serrated steak knives for cutting all foods at mealtime. Keep all knives sharpened; they are safer and easier to use than dull knives. A small salad fork also is lighter and easier to handle than a dinner fork.

☒ When eating, hold the utensil as close as possible to the tines of the fork or bowl of the spoon.

☒ Place two tight rubber bands an inch or so apart around a drinking glass. This will make it easier to grasp.

☒ Thermal mugs and children's mugs with large handles are often easier to grasp than regular glasses or cups. Insulated mugs and glasses may be used to keep drinks hot or cold without affecting the outside temperature of the glass. They are particularly useful for people who have lost sensation in their hands or have problems with coordination.

☒ If you need longer straws than those commercially available, purchase some clear tubing at a hardware store and create the length that you need.

☒ Baby plates that hold hot water help keep food warm for people who are slow in feeding themselves.

☒ Use a glass or metal pie pan instead of a regular plate if you have trouble keeping food from sliding off the plate.

☒ Use rubber circles designed to hold soap on the shower wall to help stabilize a plate. The suction cups on both sides are used. One side goes on the bottom of the plate while the other side secures the plate to the table.

☒ To get a wheelchair close to the dinner table to comfortably eat a meal, place a jelly-roll pan (a cookie sheet with sides) or a cafeteria tray lengthwise across the armrests. If these are not wide enough to rest across the armrests of your wheelchair, have someone cut a board that is the appropriate dimensions for your needs. Then push the wheelchair close to the table and allow the edge of your tray to rest flush with the edge of the table. Put your plate and drink on your new custom placemat.

☒ You can make eating easier if you elevate your plate. Experiment with different heights. Use a wicker breadbasket, a book, or a sturdy cardboard box to raise the plate to the right level.

CHAPTER 5

Personal Empowerment

When I was diagnosed with MS, I didn't know what the disease was. Yet I remember being relieved that there was a name to go with my strange, difficult-to-describe symptoms. After the initial shock of being diagnosed with a serious chronic illness wore off, the reality of it began to take hold. In the beginning the first thing for which I was unprepared was dealing with doctors, pharmacists, and therapists, and all the new medical terminology, procedures, and tests.

By nature, I'm an independent, take-charge person, so it was important for me to become an active participant in my own health care. I knew I didn't want my doctors, spouse, parents, or anyone else to "take care of me." I had rarely been to a doctor except for my pregnancies and an occasional check-up related to my job. My ob-gyn and I had an excellent relationship so I asked him to recommend an internist. I was lucky that all the doctors, (my ob-gyn, the internist, and the neurologist who diagnosed me) belonged to the same medical group so that all my medical records were in one place. Plus, there were other specialists in the group (orthopedists, physiatrists, occupational/physical/speech and language therapists) whom I could see without referrals or additional hassles with paperwork.

Over the years I have learned that a health-care provider's bedside manner is extremely important to me. If a particular doctor would not treat me with respect, listen to me, or see me as a whole person—a wife, mother, daughter, writer—I found someone who would. Learning to stick up for myself and being my own advocate has given back to me some of the power and control MS has taken away.

I also learned more than I ever wanted to know about MS. The NMSS is a wonderful resource for accurate, up-to-date information. My friends and family members also did research and collected information from newspapers, magazines, and medical journals. Some even visited the medical school library at the University of Wisconsin near my home. We shared information and learned together. It gave us something positive to do. At times I brought medical journal articles to my doctor before he or she had a chance to read them. We could discuss the findings and how they related to my case.

Here are some tips and ideas you might want to consider in managing your medical care.

I. MEDICAL ISSUES

A. Record Keeping and Research

☒ Keep a log or diary if you are experiencing new symptoms or trying a new medication. If you don't write them down, you may remember only those symptoms you actually feel when you are at your doctor's office.

☒ Begin compiling your personal medical file. The file should include past illnesses, surgical procedures, family health history, and a prescription log that includes the names and strengths of all your medications and why, when, and how often you take them. Then keep dated summaries of office appointments and copies of test results. The file will be an invaluable reference as the years pass.

☒ Get copies of all your medical records. More than half the states have enacted laws that give patients access to their hospital and physician records. Patients may have more difficulty elsewhere, but no state specifically denies access to records. The cost to obtain your medical records may vary from state to state. Keep all medical documents in a central location where they can be easily found.

☒ Summarize and keep an up-to-date, chronological list of the medical tests, treatments, surgeries, hospitalizations, and medications you have taken or are currently taking. The list does not take the place of your complete medical file. The summary gives doctors a quick overview. Then if they need more specific information they can go directly to the full report.

☒ Computer users can purchase software called Grateful Med®—The World of Medicine at Your Fingertips. The software is easy to use and provides Internet access to the world's largest medical library—the National Library of Medicine in Bethesda, Maryland. The cost is approximately $30 and gives you access to more than 8 million references. You can also ask for a layperson's overview of the illness and then graduate to the one the doctors read. For more information, contact the Office of Public Information at <http://igm.nlm.nih.gov>.

☒ Call the NMSS at (800) FIGHT MS for information about your specific type of MS. For general background on tests, procedures, or treatments, call your local NMSS chapter. You can learn to phrase your questions in the medical terms that doctors understand. You also can learn more about what symptoms you should report to your doctor.

B. Doctors' Appointments

☒ If your energy level is highest in the morning, try to get the doctor's first appointment of the day. If you do, you will be less likely to have to wait very long.

☒ Discuss how much time you will spend with the doctor at the time you make the appointment. Depending on the reason for the visit, you may be scheduled for as little as five minutes or as much as half an hour.

☒ If you are anxious to see the doctor soon, ask the receptionist if there is an earlier opening due to a cancellation. If not, ask to be notified if someone does cancel. Then call back in a few days if you have not heard from the receptionist.

☒ When you make your appointment, tell the receptionist if you will require any special help—for example, undressing or getting onto the examining table.

☒ Before leaving home, know the answers to practical questions such as: Where is there parking? What is the closest bus stop? Is there an elevator? Is the building wheelchair-accessible? Does the clinic have a wheelchair you may use?

☒ Call your doctor's office before leaving home for your appointment and ask if the doctor is running on schedule. The receptionist may suggest you come in a little later instead of spending so much time in the waiting room. Regardless of the wait time quoted over the phone, it always is wise to bring some work or a good book with you.

☒ Bring a friend or family member; between the two of you, you will remember more of what the doctor has to say about your condition and treatment options. Or tape-record your visit so you can review your doctor's explanations and answers to your questions after you get home. At the very least, you— or the person who accompanies you— should take notes of what your doctor says.

☒ The time spent with your doctor may be brief, so make the most of it by bringing a copy of your symptom diary for him or her to include in your file and preparing questions you want to ask. If you want to ask about an article you read or a report you heard on television, present as much information about it as possible. Bring a copy of the article. Make notes on the program, channel, and time of the report. With the volume of medical information available today, it is virtually impossible to know everything that is printed or said about MS.

☒ Clearly describe problems you are having without embarrassment. Be specific. If you have pain, try to describe how intense it is on a scale of 1 to 10.

☒ Share with your doctor important events in your personal, professional, and social life. Events in your life may affect your MS, and they also may affect how you take care of yourself. Learn to share this information and talk honestly about your emotions. For communication to be effective, both you and your doctor must be good listeners.

☒ Ask for an explanation, in language you can understand. Always ask your doctor to explain anything about your MS or your treatment program that you don't understand. Try repeating what you think you heard. If your physician adjusts your treatment program and you don't know why, find out the reasons for the change. Also ask about possible side effects and what you should do if they occur. Ask your doctor about side effects from medicines he or she prescribes and when the best time is to take the drug. Ask your doctor for written information about your specific type of MS.

☒ Remind doctors of previous decisions, lab results, or symptoms. Most doctors can't remember everything about you from visit to visit. If your doctor had you get lab tests before your visit, for example, ask about the results if the doctor forgets to mention them.

☒ Immediately after the appointment, go to the waiting room and look over your notes. Then if you are unclear about medication instructions, an upcoming test, or a procedure, you can ask for an explanation from the nurse before leaving the office.

☒ A nurse practitioner or physician's assistant may act as a liaison between you and the doctor. He or she can be a valuable resource for information, clarification, referral to community resources, and emotional support. Also ask if your doctor, registered nurse, or certified MS educator can help you get free samples or discounts on medical supplies. They sometimes receive promotional material or coupons.

☒ Follow your doctor's advice. If you have trouble following your treatment, talk to your doctor. Don't quit. Finding the right treatment program often involves trial and error. Be patient. Stick to proven remedies recommended by your doctor. Avoid "miracle" treatments hyped in the media or through direct advertising.

☒ Seeking a second or third opinion about a medical condition is now standard practice. To save time and expense, arm yourself with copies of your records, including test results, X-rays, and physician summaries of your condition.

C. Medications and Medical Tests

☒ Be sure to ask your doctor whether generic drugs, which are less expensive than brand-name drugs, may be used to fill your prescription. Ask if the generic drug differs from the brand-name drug in terms of efficacy. Also ask your doctor for booklets or other literature on the use and possible side effects of prescribed drugs.

☒ If you are receiving drugs from more than one doctor, no one physician will have a complete list of your medications. Avoid scattering your prescriptions among several pharmacies. Instead, pick one that fits your needs and stick to it. That way, there will be a complete record of your prescriptions and drug allergies on file in one place, and your pharmacist can easily check that a new prescription does not adversely interact with a medication you already are taking. Also find out if the medication(s) you are taking could have an adverse reaction with any over-the-counter drugs that you use. Consult the *Physician's Desk Reference* (PDR) for specific information about your medications.

☒ Before filling the prescription, get specific dosing instructions for each drug. Go over with your doctor such phrases as "three times a day" or "every eight hours." Does this mean you should take the medicine three times between 8 A.M. and bedtime, or does it literally mean every eight hours? There's a big difference. Don't assume you will find explicit instructions on the label; it may simply say "Take as directed."

☒ If you have trouble removing childproof tops from your medication bottles, your pharmacist can replace them with regular covers. However, if you have children in the house, you will need to be especially careful to store your medications safely out of children's reach. Also ask your pharmacist the best way to store medications—a high-humidity bathroom cabinet usually is the worst place to put it.

☒ Once you get home with a new medication, note on the label what the drug is for to remind you to use it only for the prescribed condition.

☒ Start a new medication as early in the day as possible. If you have an adverse reaction, it will be easier to reach the doctor.

☒ Be sure to find out what you can and cannot do to make taking your medicine easier. Is it all right to crush or break your pills—or even dissolve them in water? And is a more palatable option available, such as a liquid or granules? (It's risky simply to break open a capsule or crush a tablet. Many are *sustained-release* formulations, which are designed so that the medicine seeps into your bloodstream over many hours. To release all of the drug at once could increase your risk of side effects or could even be toxic.) If you use a medicine dropper to give liquid medications by mouth, release the liquid slowly into the cheek. Be careful not to point the dropper into the throat, which might force the medication down the windpipe. If you have difficulty swallowing a pill or tablet, place it in a teaspoon of applesauce or butter it lightly. The pill will be much easier to swallow.

☒ Order prescription refills several days in advance and ask the pharmacy to mail them to you to eliminate having to pick them up. If your medications are delivered by a courier service and you need extra time to get to the door when the delivery is made, notify the company sending you the medication of this special request when you place your order. Some companies will accommodate your request by having the delivery person wait until you answer. To have medications delivered when you aren't home, you may need to sign a release form to allow the delivery person to leave the package in a designated place.

☒ When getting a prescription refilled, ask the pharmacist to put the expiration date on the front panel of information for each prescription. Prescriptions are packaged from large bottles that contain great quantities and often are marked with an expiration date that is not transferred to monthly prescription refills.

☒ Mark on a calendar the days when medication should be increased or decreased.

☒ A seven-compartment molded plastic box with individual snap-lock compartments and a hinged lid for each compartment with a letter for each day of the week on top can be purchased at most pharmacies and makes keeping track of medications easier.

☒ If shaking down a thermometer is difficult, purchase a battery-powered thermometer with large, easy-to-read numbers. Ask your pharmacist about other devices to help you manage your home health care. For example, people who have to give themselves injections might find an auto-injector helpful. The spring-loaded device holds the syringe in position. Then all you have to do is push a button and it injects the needle into your skin.

☒ If a medication requires that you drink a large quantity of water each day, here is an easy way to keep track of your intake. Put an empty gallon container next to the sink and every time you drink a fresh glass of cold water, pour an equal amount into the gallon container. When the container is full, you know you have had the prescribed amount of water. For some people it might seem easier to fill a gallon of water, put it in the refrigerator and pour out one glass at a time, but if you can't lift and pour a water-filled container, this won't work. Using the former method enables you to avoid the strain of repeatedly lifting a heavy water jug. At the end of the day, tip the full container and gently pour the water into the sink.

D. The Hospital

☒ Before going into the hospital, ask your doctor if he or she can supply recent X-rays or lab tests so you can avoid undergoing duplicate testing at the hospital.

☒ If at all possible, avoid entering the hospital on a Friday—you might spend the weekend waiting for lab work.

☒ Make a list of phone numbers and addresses you may need while you are in the hospital. Include common numbers (those of close family and friends) as well as less common numbers (those of your next-door neighbor, landlord/manager, employer, medical supply company, and so forth). Keep this list near your bedside.

☒ Take along all the things you need from home to be comfortable. Bring in whatever you want from home, like a favorite pillow, a reacher, amplified telephone receiver, and so forth.

☒ Patients' charts can get mixed up, so talk to everyone who brings you a pill or comes to perform a test or procedure, and be sure they know who you are. That means staying alert and asking the right questions. Learn to recognize the medicines you are supposed to receive, and make sure that the person dispensing the medication checks your plastic wristband to confirm that each dose of medication is for you.

☒ You should ask about the purpose, risks, and possible discomfort of any test or procedure that is prescribed. Be clear about your needs. For example, if you have hard-to-find veins, alert the staff that you need an especially skilled person to draw your blood. If you need help getting onto the examining table, it is better to notify hospital staff in advance than to find out at the last minute that the nurse is pregnant and unable to help you.

☒ Hospitals are busy places and sometimes it is difficult to get needed rest. If you do not want to be disturbed, ask the switchboard to stop all incoming calls. Or put a "Resting, Please Do Not Disturb" sign on your door. Then if hospital personnel enter your room to pick something up or drop something off, at least they will do so quietly.

☒ If you're not up to having visitors, be honest with your friends and family when they call. In addition, you may want to put up a note on the wall above your bed that states "Please limit visits to 20 minutes" and have your doctor sign it. That way, unexpected visitors will get the message.

☒ Find out what time the nurses' shifts change so that you can ask for anything you need at least an hour before, when they aren't so busy writing up reports and performing other change-of-shift duties. In an emergency, if no one comes when you press your call button, use the bedside phone and call the hospital operator to be put through to the nurses' station.

☒ Hospitals have patient advocates—hospital employees whose job is to make sure your concerns are not overlooked. Use this resource if you are concerned that you might not be receiving adequate care. Also, if the location of the room or your roommate prevents you from getting your necessary rest, you have the right to request a transfer to another room.

☒ If you are hospitalized, it is best to designate one person to be the contact with the doctor. That way, one person is asking the questions on behalf of the family, which avoids duplication of effort by both your family members and your physician.

☒ Before you are discharged, your hospital social worker or discharge planner will want to know about your home situation. You will discuss how much care you need and who is best qualified to help you. Will someone check up on you at home on a regular basis? You will learn about community services and resources you may not be aware of that may help make the transition to home easier.

E. Managing Your Home Health Care

☒ If you have just been released from the hospital, take home the phone number of the nursing station from the floor where your room was located. Once you're home, if you have questions in the middle of the night, you will have someone to call who can allay your fears or tell you to come in for emergency treatment.

☒ If you want to keep friends and relatives apprised of your progress but don't want to be disturbed, let the answering machine provide the information. Each day record a new message updating the medical report.

☒ During the day, when children are at home, have a "quiet time" when everyone goes to his or her respective bedroom. The children do not have to nap or get into bed. Encourage reading or quiet independent play. The only rule is that children must play quietly in their room until a timer, musical alarm clock, or clock radio goes off, usually after 30 to 45 minutes. (If you set a device to go off, it takes you out of the equation and you won't be asked questions like, "Is it time to play yet? When can I come out? Why can't I go outside and play?") Children learn that when the timer goes off, they may leave their room and resume their normal activities.

☒ Use an adjustable ironing board as a bed table to hold tissues, a glass of water, reading glasses, and TV remote control.

☒ If you have trouble reading printed material such as a prescription medication insert, enlarge it. Photocopy machines at convenience store outlets, libraries, and post offices are capable of enlarging print to make it easier to read. Or use a magnifying glass to help you read.

☒ Play quiet games with your child. Board games and playing cards provide ways to interact and spend time with a child when your energy is low.

☒ As you recover from an exacerbation, your child may be "recovering," too. It is frightening for a child when Mom or Dad is sick. Sometimes a child will regress to an earlier developmental stage. However, children often regress before they make a growth spurt. Usually within 6 weeks the immature behavior will disappear and you'll see a more "mature" child.

☒ Keep a list of important telephone numbers near each telephone, such as those for police and fire departments, electric and gas companies, poison control center, family doctor, dentist, and neighbors. Make sure you have at least one telephone that does not require electricity to function so that if the power goes out but the phone lines are still up, you can make the crucial calls you need.

☒ If you need emergency medical assistance, make sure your children and neighbors know to inform the rescue workers of your condition and your special physical needs.

II. IMPROVING MEMORY AND CONCENTRATION

When I was first diagnosed with MS, cognitive problems were thought to affect only a small number of people. Today, however, it is thought that between 43 percent and 65 percent of all people with MS have some cognitive problems. Problems with concentration, memory, processing information, or communication may be very frustrating. If you think any of these thought processes have been affected, there is help. Discuss your concerns with your doctor and ask to see a psychologist, a neuropsychologist, or a speech and language therapist, who will be able to help you identify what cognitive deficits you have and how to compensate for or overcome them.

Here are some simple but effective tips to get you started.

☒ Write yourself reminder notes and put them where you will be sure to see them. For example, put a Post-It™ note on the door to the garage to remind you to stop at the post office for stamps or on your bathroom mirror to remind you to call to wish a friend a happy birthday.

☒ Buy a small spiral notebook and a small pen or pencil that you can stick in the spiral binding. Keep the notebook in your purse. Or wear a gardener's apron in the house because it has generous front pockets. Keep your notebook and pencil in one of the pockets.

☒ If you like gadgets, purchase an electronic pocket organizer and use it to keep your address and appointment books, notes, and to-do lists.

☒ Use a timer or alarm clock that you have to physically turn off, as opposed to one that rings only once, as a reminder to turn on the oven to start dinner.

☒ Have your computer "beep" to remind you to take a break and put your feet up. Program your pager with reminders, such as when to take your medications, move the sprinkler in the yard, or perform certain job-related tasks.

☒ To remember to take a medication first thing in the morning, put the pill bottle in your slipper. Before you can put on your slippers, you must remove the pill bottle.

☒ For tasks that have no definite ending time, put an old bracelet around your wrist when you begin the task to remind you that it needs to be finished. Put the bracelet on when you begin, for example, watering the yard or simmering soup in a stockpot. If you lose track of time, the bracelet will remind you to return to the task. When you're finished, take the bracelet off and put it around the faucet or next to the stove so it's ready to use the next time.

☒ If it's an inopportune or inconvenient time to write yourself a note, like in a darkened movie theater or out walking the dog, take off a ring and put it on different finger, put your watch on the "wrong" wrist, or double knot your shoelaces. That way, you'll be reminded of the task and can make a note of it at a more convenient time.

☒ If you're "musical," create a little melody to help you remember a telephone number or sequence of steps.

☒ No paper handy to write down things you need to remember? Try this: create a word from the first letter of each item on your list. C-R-O-W for example, might mean: **C**all for airline tickets, **R**eturn library books, **O**rder birthday cake, **W**ater plants.

☒ Use an audiocassette tape player to record daily tasks.

☒ If you have trouble remembering whether or not you have done a task—for example, locking the door when you leave the house—try this: say out loud, "I'm locking the door" as you lock up, and see if that helps.

☒ Think over the route for the stops on your errand trips and write it down if you are prone to forgetting the sequence. Before you leave home, consider: Is this a good time of day to be going to the library or post office? Will the drive-up windows at the bank be open? Will there be lines? Rearrange the sequence of stops to make it most convenient for you.

☒ Women can use the flap of a saddlebag purse as a "note board." Using plain white, self-adhesive mailing labels, write notes on them, peel the labels off their backing, and stick them on the inside of the foldover flap of the purse. Once a task or errand has been completed, peel off the label and toss it out.

☒ When you are out and about and want to remember to do something when you return home, call yourself and leave a message on your answering machine.

☒ If remembering and writing down numbers quickly presents a problem, keep a calculator near the phone and use it to write down a number left on the answering machine.

☒ Use a calculator with a paper tape to add long sequences of numbers. Then you can recheck your work for skipped or transposed numbers.

☒ Say the numbers out loud and see if that improves your ability to add and subtract numbers in your checkbook. Or consider using a money-management computer software program that does the math for you.

☒ At large gatherings like weddings, reunions, parties, and other special events, the noise and room activity may make following conversations difficult. Ask if you may move to

a quieter, less frenetic area, such as a lobby
or patio, to continue a conversation.

III. QUIET RESTFUL ACTIVITIES

A. Reading

☒ Make sure you get needed rest. If you enjoy
reading, you may find that new books sometimes are stiff and difficult to keep open.
Have someone "break the spine" of the book
by opening up pages and flattening the
pages at several different parts of the book.
Or purchase used books, which are worn
and not as stiff as new books.

☒ To turn pages in a book, use the eraser on a
pencil or a rubber fingertip like those used
by secretaries and bookkeepers.

☒ You may reserve library books by calling the
library or using the library's Internet connection. Then the library will let you know
when the reserved books are in and ready
for pickup. Some communities have volun-
teers who will drop off and pick up library
books at no charge.

☒ Take advantage of the library's collection of
large-print and audio books. The *Large-Type
Books in Print* directory has more than 3,000
entries and includes books and periodicals
published in large print. This reference book
is available at most major libraries.

The Book Clubs division of Doubleday & Company has a large-print home library. A wide range of full-length hardcover best-sellers, including fiction, mystery, romance, and how-to titles, are offered. For more information, call (800) 343-4300.

If you have a documented physical or visual disability, you may qualify for the National Library Service for the Blind and Physically Handicapped Talking Book Program. These books are sent and returned by mail postage-free. The books require a special tape player, which is loaned to you free of charge.

☒ Find out if your local radio stations broadcast readings from novels. Stations often have a program where a chapter is read from a current novel each day.

☒ Make reading while lying flat in bed easier with Bed Specs or Prism glasses. You wear them just like a regular pair of glasses (they may even be worn over your existing glasses), and they allow you to see a book or television screen even when you are lying on your back. They may be adjusted to any head width. Contact Maddak Inc. at 6 Industrial Rd., Pequannock, NJ 07440-1993, (973) 628-7600, fax (973) 305-0841.

B. Watching Television

☒ If your current remote controls are too difficult to operate, replace them with a single "universal" remote, which controls your TV, stereo, and VCR. You can find universal remotes where TVs and electronic devices are sold.

☒ Take a plain adhesive-backed label and write the cable channels and their numbers on it. Then put the label on the back of your remote control so you don't have to remember all the numbers or page through a TV program schedule to find what you want to watch.

☒ Keep remote controls, TV program schedules, reading glasses, pens, and paper within easy reach wherever you sit by using an adjustable hospital bed table. Or create your own saddlebag-style holder for your TV and VCR remote control devices. Select two hand towels that will fit your decor and room colors and sew them together at one end to make one long piece. Then fold up each end, creating pockets to hold your remotes. If possible, divide one of the pockets in half and use it to hold a pencil and notepad. You also may want to secure your holder to the arm of your couch or chair with a few stitches.

C. Playing Games

☒ Jumbo playing cards are available at many drugstores and are easier to use than regular cards. To make it easier to hold cards, take an old shoebox, remove the top, and put the bottom of the box inside the cover. The space between the cover and the side of the shoebox holds the cards nicely.

☒ A revolving game board compensates for limited reach in such games as Parcheesi™, Scrabble™, or jigsaw puzzles. You can purchase your own base and put a piece of plywood on the turntable or use a kitchen Lazy Susan for turning the game board.

☒ If you have trouble handling game pieces, substitute larger items like Lego™ blocks, empty plastic pill bottles, or little plastic finger puppets. To adapt game pieces like those that come with games such as Candyland™, glue a piece of cardboard on the bottom to make the base slightly larger.

IV. WEEKEND GETAWAYS AND EXTENDED TRAVEL

A change of scenery may be the pick-me-up we all need. However, for people living with MS, changing daily routines and leaving the comforts of home may be a little scary. But with a little pre-planning and a spirit of adventure, travelers with special needs may enjoy a weekend getaway or a major family vacation just like everyone else. Here are some tips to make your travel easier. Bon voyage!

A. Preparing for Your Trip

☒ Here's a no-hassle way to get ready for family trips and vacations: make three lists.

The first list should contain the obvious—clothing, accessories, toiletries, and so forth—and the not so obvious—trip information (maps, itinerary, passport), address book, stamps for postcards, laundry bag (for dirty clothes), extra canvas bag (for purchases), and "fun stuff" (games, reading material, sporting equipment).

The second list should include chores that may be done a few days before you leave: Get substitute drivers for carpools. Cancel lessons. Find someone to mow the lawn (or shovel the snow). Arrange for newspaper and mail pick-up. Leave a key and itinerary (with phone numbers) with neighbors. For car trips, add: Check air in the tires (including the spare). Purchase snack foods for the cooler. Put selected tools in the trunk in case of an emergency.

The third list should include things to do immediately before you leave: Set timer lights. Turn down thermostat and hot water heater. Grind anything left in the garbage disposal and take out the garbage. Check to see that electric blankets, curling iron, stove, oven, and coffee maker are turned off. And, finally, check to see that all the doors and windows are locked.

☒ To obtain information about an unfamiliar destination, contact the Convention and Visitors' Bureau of the state you will visit or the Chamber of Commerce of the city of interest. These offices can send you brochures and give you information on attractions, accommodations, restaurants, and so on. Be sure to find a motel or hotel that is centrally located to the areas you plan to visit because you don't want to waste time and energy traveling from one side of town to another.

☒ If you have vision problems and reading highway maps is difficult, take maps of your route and destination to a copy shop and have them enlarged for easier reading.

☒ Before making a trip to a new destination, contact the hotel concierge and ask that he or she put together a packet of tourist information for the dates of your visit. With that information, you can make restaurant reservations, arrange for theater tickets, and schedule the sights that you want to see.

B. Traveling By Car

☒ When traveling by car to an unfamiliar location, plot your route and mark it on the map with a highlighter pen. Or write down the directions. Designate a navigator and a map reader. It usually is easy to read highway maps. However, when you get to metropolitan areas, it may be nearly impossible to read the small print on street maps, especially in a moving car. To solve this problem, enlarge the street map a couple of times on a photocopying machine at your neighborhood library or copy shop.

☒ When you consult a road map and choose your route, fold the map into a 5 inch x 5

inch square, making your entire route
visible. Then put a paper clip on the "north"
edge of the map. This will make it easier for
the navigator to handle the map and keep
the orientation correct.

☒ Keep a magnifying glass with a light on it in
the glove compartment of your car. This will
come in handy when you need to consult a
map.

☒ When traveling on unfamiliar interstate
highways, here is a way to determine
whether an exit off the highway would be
to the right or to the left. The small exit
panels on the tops of road signs indicate
which side the exit is on. If the small panel
is on the right side of the sign, it's a right
lane exit ramp. If it's on the left side, it's a
left lane exit ramp. Another fact to
remember is that on the interstate highway
system odd-numbered roads go north and
south while even-numbered roads go east
and west.

☒ When you travel, take along your personal
disabled windshield placard. Disabled
parking permits are honored in most states
and you may use the placard on a rental car
or in a car in which you are a passenger. If
you forget to bring your permit with you,
your only option may be to visit the nearest
Motor Vehicle Department office and request
a temporary permit. Don't be surprised if
they want to see a doctor's letter certifying
your disability or medical condition.

☒ If you travel by car with children, take along a jump rope, Frisbee™, balls, roller skates, or other toys they can use to work off excess energy when you stop at rest areas.

C. Air Travel

☒ With heightened airport security, passengers must present a photo ID—usually a driver's license—when checking in so that airport personnel can match your picture ID with the name on the ticket. If you do not have a driver's license because you are unable to drive, call your state's Department of Motor Vehicles to find out how to obtain a state picture identification card. You may have to turn in your expired driver's license for a picture ID, and there might be a small service charge. If you don't have an expired license, you will need a certified copy of your birth certificate or a passport and a copy of your signature on a document such as a contract or tax return. Specific require-ments differ from state to state.

☒ If you're traveling on an airline flight on which a meal will be served and you need a vegetarian, low-salt, kosher, or other special meal, be sure to contact the airline at least 48 hours in advance of your flight.

☒ When you reach the airport, do not hesitate to take advantage of the services available to travelers. Check your luggage with an airline representative at the curb instead of hauling it to the counter, or ask a porter to carry it for you. Once inside, avoid a long, tiring walk through crowded corridors by requesting transport to your flight gate on a motorized cart or by requesting a wheelchair. The agent at the ticket counter can call for a wheelchair for you to use while you're in the airport.

☒ When you check in at the ticket counter at the airport, request a seat without a seatmate. If there are empty seats, the ticket agent will be happy to change your seat assignment. Bulkhead seats on airplanes may offer the extra space a traveler with a disability needs. However, bulkhead seats rarely have lift-up armrests, which could be even more helpful to some travelers with special needs. When selecting seat assignments, ask the ticket agent about the options available on your plane.

☒ If you are worried about being disturbed on a long airline flight by passengers using the on-board facilities, sit as far away from the restrooms as possible. Ask the flight attendant for a blanket and pillow as soon as you're seated. A plane often does not have enough room to carry blankets and pillows for every passenger.

☒ If you travel by air with an electric wheelchair, scooter, or other important piece of equipment, tag all parts with your name, address, and telephone number so they will not get lost if the equipment must be disassembled to fit into the cargo hold. As an added safety precaution, take along a copy of the assembly instructions in case you need it when you arrive at your destination.

☒ If you use a three-wheeled scooter or wheelchair, traveling by air is straightforward but does require a bit of planning. At most airports you will be boarded before other passengers and may take your own chair or scooter to the door of the plane. Your companion or a porter will help you transfer to an "aisle chair" that can navigate the narrow airplane aisle. Once on the plane, your companion or the employee will assist you out of the aisle chair and into a seat. If you have a manual folding wheelchair, it will be stowed at your request in a closet in the cabin on any plane that has adequate storage, and has priority over any other baggage. Otherwise, it will be taken from the jetway into the hold; be sure to get the special door-tag ticket issued to make sure your wheelchair is delivered back to the jetway at your destination. When you arrive, passengers needing assistance must wait until others are off the plane. Then you can leave the plane on the aisle chair. Your scooter or wheelchair will be waiting for you in the jetway. Have your companion or airline personnel help you out of the aisle chair into your scooter and you're off!

☒ When you travel great distances by air with medications that must be refrigerated, carry a cooler with you on the plane. Keep ice cubes in the cooler in a sealed plastic bag.

When the ice melts, pour out the water and ask the flight attendant for more ice.

D. Foreign Travel

☒ If you are traveling overseas, take a photocopy of your passport and two passport photos with you and keep them separate from your passport. Then if your passport is lost or stolen, you will have what you need to replace it.

E. Packing

☒ Travel light. Purchase trial-size bottles and tubes of everything from shampoo and hair spray to toothpaste and mouthwash, or purchase empty travel-size bottles that you can fill with your own toiletries. It's amazing how much lighter your suitcase will be.

☒ Carry all your medications and other absolute necessities in your carry-on bag, so if your checked luggage is lost or misplaced you will still have what you need on hand.

☒ Both you and your traveling companion should pack a change of clothes in each other's luggage in case one of the bags is lost or delayed.

☒ For comfort on the go, take a special pillow from home because it may help you sleep better. It's hard to get comfortable if the pillow isn't "right."

☒ Take a bed jacket or robe to wear if the room is chilly and you're waiting for the heat to kick in.

☒ Extra blankets and pillows usually are available by calling the front desk of a hotel or motel.

☒ Pack a bent-neck straw to make drinking a glass of water easier while lying in bed.

☒ Take along a free-standing mirror that can rest on a table, counter, or nightstand. Mirrors often are difficult to get close to, especially for people who use a wheelchair.

☒ Take a soap-on-a-rope. It eliminates the need to hold onto a slippery bar of soap in an unfamiliar shower where the soap dish and grab rails may not be located where you need them.

☒ Take along a portable smoke alarm.

☒ Pack a second pair of eyeglasses.

☒ Stay at hotels or motels that have laundry facilities for guests. You can pack less. Purchase trial sizes of laundry detergent or fill travel bottles with your own supply of detergent and pack them in your suitcase.

F. Staying at a Motel or Hotel

☒ If you're not sure where to stay, rely on travel agents to guide you in making your plans. There usually is no charge for their services. In fact, you often will save money because travel agents know about special rates and weekend packages. Whether you make the reservations yourself or work with a travel agent, always be completely honest about your needs. Some specialized travel agencies now focus on the needs of travelers with disabilities. See the resource section for information.

☒ If you make hotel or motel reservations through a toll-free number, be aware that the operator will not be able to answer your specific accessibility questions. You will have to call the motel or hotel directly. If you want a "handicapped" room, ask how you can ensure that the room will be held until you arrive.

☒ Accessibility standards vary from state to state, but in general newly constructed or recently remodeled buildings have the best facilities for disabled travelers. Older motels or hotels may or may not be accessible. Always ask about accommodations when making your reservations.

☒ Most, if not all, motels or hotels have "handicapped" rooms. These rooms are available to all guests, regardless of their disability. Accessible rooms are either larger than regular rooms or have less furniture in them, so they have more room to walk or wheel around in. The rooms generally have extra-large bathrooms with a raised toilet and grab bars by the toilet and inside the tub and/or shower. Sometimes there is a fold-down seat in the shower stall. (If there is no shower seat, ask if they have a shower chair you may use during your stay.) Light switches usually are lower and doorway openings are wider. In addition to regular smoke alarms, accessible rooms often have flashing lights to alert hearing-impaired guests in case of fire. If walking stairs is a problem, request a room on a lower floor near stairways and exits. Remember that elevators may not be used in a fire emergency.

☒ Some travelers may find that the "suite" concept makes traveling easier. In all-suites hotels, guests have a two-room suite consisting of a sitting room and a bedroom. The sitting room usually has a couch that converts to a queen-sized bed, a table and chairs, a telephone, a TV set, and a kitchen area with a microwave, refrigerator, and wet bar. The bedroom may have another telephone and a TV with a remote control. Generally, the bathroom is off the hallway that separates the two rooms. Complimentary breakfast may be served, and guests are encouraged to bring snack foods and beverages to keep in their rooms.

☒ For a long weekend or an extended stay, travelers may want to stay at a residence motel or hotel. Each "room" usually has a fully equipped kitchen, including a stove, refrigerator, dishwasher, garbage disposal, pots, pans, dishes, and so on. Some chains have a grocery shopping service for guests and will fill the cabinets and refrigerator with items they request. Some serve a continental breakfast each morning. The suite and inn concepts are wonderful for travelers who have special needs. While someone naps in the bedroom, others may watch TV, play cards, read a book, and so on. In addition, those who need to refrigerate medication or carefully monitor their diet will find the microwave and refrigerator more of a necessity than a convenience.

G. Out and About

☒ Use a wheelchair when you want to visit a zoo, a museum, an art gallery, or a historic monument. Conserve energy and you will see more sights and have more new adventures. If fatigue is a problem, you may want to rent a wheelchair to take with you. Rental wheelchairs are available from pharmacies, medical supply companies, or rental stores. Check and compare their prices and services.

☒ Carry trail mix, nuts, and/or fresh fruit with you. Eat a healthy snack and avoid the temptation to grab a candy bar with hollow calories and little nutritional value.

☒ Take an adequate supply of prescription medications with you, and don't forget any over-the-counter remedies that you might need (buying them on the road in travel sizes or from hotel gift shops often is very expensive). You may want to carry a doctor's

prescription in your wallet or have your prescriptions filled at a pharmacy that uses a
computer network. If you are delayed for
some reason, you can have your prescription
refilled. Take the prescription for your eyeglasses, as well. If they are lost or damaged,
you usually can have a replacement pair
made in a short time. Also take along your
doctor's phone number. That way, if there's a
problem filling the prescription or you have
a medical emergency or problem on the trip,
you will be able to contact your doctor
easily.

☒ If you are traveling with children, have each
child over the age of 3 years take along a
backpack or book bag with his or her own
toys, books, games, and so forth. Let them
make their own decisions about what to
pack. The only rule should be that they must
be able to carry their filled bags themselves.

H. Travel Resources

☒ The International Association for Medical
Assistance to Travelers (417 Center Street,
Lewiston, NY 14092, (716) 754-4883) is a
nonprofit organization that provides important information to travelers with medical
concerns. Travelers can obtain a directory of
English-speaking doctors in foreign countries. Updated each year, the directory lists
doctors who have had training in the United
States, Great Britain, or Canada. IAMA also
has world immunization charts, malaria risk
charts, and world climate charts, and can

tell you about the food and water in the countries you plan to visit.

☒ The International Association of Convention & Visitor Bureaus (2000 L St. NW, Suite 702, Washington, D.C. 20036-4990; (202) 296-7888; fax (202) 296-7889; *<info@iacvb. org;*info@iacvb.org>; *<http://www.iacvb.org* http://www.iacvb.org>) publishes a free directory listing the telephone numbers and fax numbers for convention and visitor bureaus for large cities all over the world. Try calling the travel and tourist information bureau of the state you're planning to visit for information on accessibility. Better yet, call the tourism office of the county or city of your destination to find accessible attractions and lodgings. Be persistent.

If you're still apprehensive about leaving familiar surroundings, become a member of the Travelin' Talk Network, (P.O. Box 3534, Clarksville, TN 37043-3534, (931) 552-6670). It's a valuable resource for travelers with special needs. Members of the network share knowledge of their hometowns and/or extend a multitude of services to travelers who need help. Whether your wheelchair breaks down or you're trying to locate an accessible vegetarian restaurant, Travelin' Talk members are "your friends away from home." Membership is on a sliding scale, with $10 the maximum individual contribution. The founder, Rick Crowder, recently published a directory listing Travelin' Talk members all over the world ($35). In addition, he publishes a quarterly newsletter that includes the names and locations of new members, travel tips, and stories of the ways people are helping each other.

CHAPTER 6

Additional Resources for People with Multiple Sclerosis

T here is a vast array of resources available to help make life easier while living with MS. The following is a selection of useful references.

Information Sources

Information Center and Library, National Multiple Sclerosis Society (733 Third Avenue, New York, NY 10017; tel: (800) FIGHT MS). The Center will answer questions and send you publications of the Society as well as copies of published articles on any topics related to MS.

Accent on Information (P.O. Box 700, Bloomington, IL 61702; tel: (304) 378-2961). A computerized retrieval system of information for the disabled about problems relating to activities of daily living and home management. There is a small charge for a basic search and photocopies, but people with disabilities who are unable to pay are never denied services.

Electronic Information Sources

Some of these sources of information are available only if you are a subscriber to the service. However, there are also many sources of information available free through the Internet on the World Wide Web. For example, the National Multiple Sclerosis Society has a home page on the World Wide Web at: <http://www.nmss.org>. The other sources of MS information on the World Wide Web are too numerous to list. If you are an experienced "net surfer," switch to your favorite search engine and enter the key words "MS" or "multiple sclerosis." This will generally give you a listing of dozens of web sites that pertain to MS. Keep in mind, however, that the World Wide Web is a free and open medium; while many of the web sites have excellent and useful information, others may contain highly unusual and inaccurate information.

- *America OnLine*: (800) 827-6364 (GO TO NMSS).
- *CompuServe*: (800) 487-6227 (GO MULTSCLER).
- *Prodigy*: (800) 776-3449 (JUMP MS FORUM).

On the Internet: Access <USENET NEWS-GROUP-ALT.SUPPORT.MULT-SCLEROSIS>.

Books

The Complete Directory for People with Disabilities, 1997/98 edition. Includes organizations and associations that serve people with all types of disabilities along with their phone numbers, addresses, and contact names. There is also a chapter on more than 700 assistive devices covering everything from automotive aids to bath aids to games and toys for children. Information on rehabilitation centers, job training programs, computer centers and devices, and camps. It provides a wealth of resources for people with disabilities. Also, finally, a fully annotated descriptive bibliography of more than 600 books and professional texts that are new to the market and will make sure that the user has the best current information available. (832 pages, Paperback, $145.00, ISBN: 0-939300-86-9; Hard cover, $170.00, ISBN: 0-939300-95-8. Edited by L. Mackenzie, published by Grey House Publishing Inc., Pocket Knife Square, Lakeville, CT 06039; phone (860)435-0808; fax (860) 435-0867; <www.greyhouse.com; book@greyhouse.com>). Your local library may have a copy of this reference book.

Living with Low Vision: A Resource Guide for People with Sight Loss. (Resources for Rehabilitation, 33 Bedford Street, Suite 19A, Lexington, MA 02173; tel: (617)862-6455). The only large print comprehensive guide to services and products designed to assist individuals with vision loss throughout North America.

Resources for People with Disabilities and Chronic Conditions. (Resources for Rehabilitation, 33 Bedford Street, Suite 19A, Lexington, MA 02173; tel: (617) 862-6455). A comprehensive resource guide covering a variety of disabling conditions as well as general information on rehabilitation services, assistive technology for independent living, and laws that affect people with disabilities.

Resource Directory for the Disabled. (Written by R.N. Shrout, published by Facts-on-File, 460 Park Avenue South, New York, NY 10016, 1991). A resource directory that includes associations and organizations, government agencies, libraries and research centers, publications, and products of all types for disabled individuals.

Agencies and Organizations

ABLEDATA Database (tel: (800) 227-0216, <http://www.abledata.com/database.htm>) currently lists more than 24,000 products from nearly 3,000 domestic and international manufacturers and distributors. The database is indexed according to product type. Products listed may be commercially available, one-of-a-kind or prototype devices, custom adaptations of commercially available products, or do-it-yourself devices.

Disabilities Resources Monthly Newsletter and DRM WebWatcher (Disability Resources, Inc.,

Dept. IN< Four Glatter Lane, Centereach, NY 11720-1032. Call or fax (516) 585-0290, <jklauber@disability resources.org> or <http://@suffolk,lib.ny,us>, <http://www.disabili-tyresources.org>, or <http://www.geocities.com/-drm>) feature several hundred topics and disability resources. Books, documents, databases, and other informational materials of national or international interest are briefly described and cross-referenced to related subjects.

National Multiple Sclerosis Society (NMSS) (733 Third Avenue, New York, NY 10017; tel: (800) FIGHT MS). The NMSS funds both basic and health services research. An office of professional education programs maintains a speakers' bureau and supports professional education programs in the individual chapters. Chapters and branches of the Society provide direct services to people with MS and their families, including information and referral, counseling, equipment loan, and social and recreational support programs. The National Office will put you in touch with your closest chapter. The Information Center and Library is available to answer questions and provide a wide range of educational materials, as well as reprints of articles written about MS.

National Rehabilitation Information Center (NARIC) (8455 Colesville Road, Suite 935, Silver Spring, MD, 20910-3319; tel: (800) 346-2742 or (301) 588-9284, TTY (301) 495-5626, fax: (301) 587-1967, <http://www.naric.com/naric/index.html>). An organization serving anyone, professional or layperson, who is interested in disability and reha-bilitation, including consumers, family members, health professionals, educators, rehabilitation counselors, students, librarians, administrators, and researchers.

Paralyzed Veterans of America (PVA) (801 Eighteenth Street N.W., Washington, D.C. 20006; tel: (800) 424-8200). PVA is a national information and advocacy agency working to restore function and quality of life for veterans with spinal cord dysfunction. It supports and funds education and research and has a national advocacy program that focuses on accessibility issues. PVA publishes brochures on many issues related to rehabilitation.

Eastern Paralyzed Veterans Association (EPVA) (75-20 Astoria Boulevard, Jackson Heights, NY 11370; tel: (718) 803-EPVA). EPVA is a private, nonprofit organization dedicated to serving the needs of its members as well as other people with disabilities. While offering a wide range of benefits to member veterans with spinal cord dysfunction (including hospital liaison, sports and recreation, wheelchair repair, adaptive architectural consultations, research and educational services, communications, and library and information services, they will also provide brochures and information on a variety of subjects, free of charge to the general public.

Health Resource Center for Women with Disabilities (Rehabilitation Institute of Chicago, Chicago, IL 60612; tel: (312) 908-7997). The Center is a project run by and for women with disabilities. It publishes a free newsletter, "Resourceful Women," and offers support groups and educational seminars addressing issues from a disabled woman's perspective. Among its many educational resources, the Center has developed a video on mothering with a disability.

Assistive Technology

Access to Recreation: Adaptive Recreation Equipment for the Physically Challenged (2509 E. Thousand Oaks Boulevard, Suite 430, Thousand Oaks, CA 91362; tel: (800) 634-4351). Products include exercise equipment and assistive devices for sports, environmental access, games, crafts, and hobbies.

adaptABILITY (Department 2082, Norwich Avenue, Colchester, CT 06415; tel: (800) 243-9232). A free catalog of assistive devices and self-care equipment designed to enhance independence.

Enrichments (P.O. Box 5050, Bolingbrook, IL 60440; tel: (800) 323-5547). A free catalog of assistive devices and self-care equipment designed to enhance independence.

Sears Home Health Care Catalog (P.O. Box 3123, Naperville, IL 60566; tel: (800) 326-1750). The catalog includes medical equipment such as hospital beds, commodes, and wheelchairs, as well as adaptive clothing.

Environmental Adaptations

A Consumer's Guide to Home Adaptation (Adaptive Environments Center, 374 Congress Street, Suite 301, Boston, MA 02210; tel: (617) 695-1225).

A workbook for planning adaptive home modifications such as lowering kitchen countertops and widening doorways.

"Adapting the Home for the Physically Challenged" (A/V Health Services, P.O. Box 1622, West Sacramento, CA 95691; tel: (703)389-4339). A 22-minute videotape that describes home modifications for individuals who use walkers or wheelchairs. Ramp construction and room modification specifications are included.

National Kitchen and Bath Association (687 Willow Grove Street, Hackettstown, NJ 07840; tel: (908)852-0033). The Association produces a technical manual of barrier-free planning and has directories of certified designers and planners.

GE Answer Center (9500 Williamsburg Plaza, Louisville, KY 40222; tel: (800)626-2000). The Center, which is open twenty-four hours a day, seven days a week, offers assistance to individuals with disabilities as well as the general public. They offer two free brochures, "Appliance Help for Those with Special Needs" and "Basic Kitchen Planning for the Physically Handicapped."

Travel

Information for Handicapped Travelers (available free of charge from the National Library Service for the Blind and Physically Handicapped, 1291 Taylor Street, N.W., Washington, D.C. 20542; tel: (800)424-8567; (202)707-5100). A booklet providing information about travel agents, transportation, and information centers for individuals with disabilities.

Society for the Advancement of Travel for the Handicapped (SATH) (347 Fifth Avenue, Suite 610, New York, NY 10016; tel: (212)447-7284). SATH is a nonprofit organization that acts as a clearinghouse for accessible tourism information and is in contact with organizations in many countries to promote the development of facilities for disabled people. SATH publishes a quarterly magazine, "Access to Travel."

Travel for the Disabled: A Handbook of Travel Resources and 500 Worldwide Access Guides. (Written by Helen Hecker, published by Twin Peaks Press, P.O. Box 129, Vancouver, WA 98666; tel: (800)637-2256). The handbook provides information for disabled travelers about accessibility.

Access-Able Travel Source, a free Internet information service for travelers with disabilities, can be contacted at P.O. Box 1796, Wheat Ridge, CO 80034, (303) 232-2929, or directly on the Internet at www.access-able.com.

Travelin' Talk (P.O. Box 3534, Clarksville, TN 37043; tel: (615)552-6670). A network of more than 1,000 people and organizations around the world who are willing to provide assistance to travelers with disabilities and share their knowledge about the areas in which they live. Travelin' Talk publishes a newsletter by the same name and has an extensive resource directory.

Visual Impairment

The Lighthouse Low Vision Products Consumer Catalog (36-20 Northern Boulevard, Long Island City, NY 11101; tel: (800)829-0500). This large-print catalog offers a wide range of products designed to help people with impaired vision.

The Library of Congress, Division for the Blind and Physically Handicapped (1291 Taylor Street, N.W., Washington, D.C. 20542; tel: (800)424-8567; (800)424-9100; for application: (202)287-5100). The Library Service provides free talking book equipment on loan as well as a full range of recorded books for individuals with disabilities or visual impairment. It also provides a variety of free library services through 140 cooperating libraries.

Speech Impairment

Attainment Co. Inc., P.O. Box 930160, Verona WI 53593-0160. Provides a simple and inexpensive device to assist people with speech impairment.

Publishing Companies Specializing in Health and Disability Issues

Demos Medical Publishing (386 Park Avenue South, Suite 201, New York, NY 10016; tel: (800) 532-8663).

Resources for Rehabilitation (33 Bedford Street, Suite 19A, Lexington, MA 02173; tel: (617)862-6455).

Woodbine House (Publishers of the Special-Needs Collection) (6510 Bells Mill Road, Bethesda, MD 20817; tel: (301)897-3570; (800)843-7323).

☒ Purchase postage stamps by mail at no extra cost. "The Easy Stamp—Stamps by Mail" service is available throughout the United States. Simply call your local post office or ask your letter carrier for an order blank. There's no minimum order and stamps are delivered to you within three to five business days.

☒ If your mail is delivered to a mailbox at the curb or at the mouth of your driveway and you have a documented physical or medical problem, you may qualify to have your mail delivered directly to your door. Known as a "hardship delivery," this service is available by submitting a written request with appropriate documentation to your local postmaster. If your request is denied and you want to appeal the decision, contact the Consumer Advocate, U.S. Postal Service, 475 L'Enfant Plaza, Washington, DC 20260-6320.

☒ Several nonprofit organizations provide specially trained service dogs to individuals with mobility impairments. These dogs can be trained to respond to about 90 commands, and they help with day-to-day activities such as retrieving dropped items or items on shelves, opening doors, pulling wheelchairs up ramps, turning on lights, and assisting with counter exchanges at banks and stores. Assistance dog services match an individual dog with an individual person, taking into account the abilities and temperaments of both parties. Call the Assistance Dog United Campaign at (800) 248-DOGS (3647) for information on how to obtain a service dog. Also check out the Service-dogs Internet listserv by sending a message with a blank subject line to *<major-domo@acpub.duke.edu>* with the following words in the body of the message: subscribe service-dogs. You can send messages to the list at *<service-dogs@acpub.duke.edu>*.

About the Author

Shelley Peterman Schwarz and her husband, Dave, live in Madison, Wisconsin. They have been married since 1969 and are enjoying the sounds of the "Empty Nest Symphony." Their daughter, Jamie, graduated from the University of Wisconsin School of Business and works in Chicago. Their son, Andy, is a student at the University of Wisconsin, studying environmental engineering.

At the time of her diagnosis in 1979, Shelley was working part-time as a teacher of the deaf. In 1985, when a story she wrote appeared in *Inside MS,* the magazine of the NMSS, a new career was born. Since then Shelley has published more than 350 articles and received numerous awards including the *Mother of the Year* from the Wisconsin Chapter of the National MS Society, the *Partner in Health* award from the Combined Health Appeal of America, and the *Spirit of the American Woman* award from J.C. Penney.

Shelley's syndicated "Making Life Easier" column appears in numerous newspapers and magazines across the country, including *Inside MS, Real Living with MS, Enable,* and *Friendly Wheels* magazines, to name just a few. In 1997 the National Arthritis Foundation, Inc. commissioned Shelley to write *250 Tips for Making Life with Arthritis Easier* based on her "Making Life Easier" column. Shelley has also self-published three books. They are *The Best 25 Catalog Resources for Making Life Easier* (updated 1998), *Dressing Tips and Clothing Resources for Making Life Easier* (updated and expanded 1998), and *Blooming Where You're Planted: Stories from the Heart* (1998).

Shelley also is a professional speaker and a member of the National Speaker's Association. Her philosophy of life is to find solutions to whatever problems she faces and to help others do the same. Her motivational and inspirational keynotes and workshops help audiences see challenges in their lives as opportunities for personal growth. She shares her message of hope and teaches audiences how to "bloom wherever they're planted."

Index

Accessibility
  hotels and motels and,
    84–85
  kitchen and, 40–42
  public accommodations
    and, 6
Accessories, clothing, 38
Adaptive devices, for
    mealtime, 48–50
Air travel, 79–82
Airline meals, 79
Alterations, clothing, 30–32
Ankle-foot-orthosis, 33

Bagging groceries, 47
Bath mat, 14–15
Bathing, 26
Bathing children, 27
Bathroom, safety and
    accessibility, 14–16
Bathtub adaptations, 14–15
Bedding, 17
Bedroom, safety and
    accessibility, 16–18
Boots, 30

Bulkhead seats, air travel
    and, 80
Button hook, 31
Buttonholes, 31

Carpeting, 18
Cast, dressing with, 29
Casters, furniture and, 18
Catalog shopping, 35
Chairs, 18
Childproof tops,
    medications and,
    59–60
Children
  bathing, 27
  dressing, 30
  "quiet time" and, 66
  traveling with, 87
Closets, bedroom, 17–18
Clothing alterations, 30–32
Cognitive problems, 67–72
Computers and technology,
    20–23
Cotton clothing, 35
Cutting board, 42

105

Decals, tub and shower, 14
Dental floss, 27
Dimmer light switch, 9
Disabled windshield
    placard, 78
Doctors' appointments,
    54–58
Doorknobs, 10–12
Doors, 10–12
Doorways, 10–12
Dosing instructions,
    medications and, 59
Dressing children, 30
Dressing in layers, 29
Dressing stick, 29
Dressing tips, 28–30
Dycem™, 42

Earrings, 37
Elastic thread, buttons and,
    31
Expiration dates,
    prescription medication
    and, 61
Extended travel, 75–87

Faucets, 13–14
Fire precautions, 9
Flashlight, use of at night, 17
Footwear, 32–34
  shopping for, 37
Foreign travel, 82
Furniture, 18

Game-playing, 74–75
Garage door openers, 12
General tips, 1–6
Generic drugs, 58
Grab bars, 12–13, 15
Grateful Med®, 43

Grocery carts, 5
Grocery shopping, 5, 46–48
Grooming, 26–28

Handles, for combs and
    brushes, 27
Highway maps, vision
    problems and, 77
Home health care, 65–67
Home office, 20–23
Home safety and
    accessibility, 8–20
  bathroom, 14–16
  bedroom, 16–18
  doorknobs, doors, and
    doorways, 10–12
  faucets and sinks, 13–14
  furniture and rugs, 18
  housecleaning, 18–19
  laundry, 19–20
  lighting and light
    switches, 9–10
  locks and keys, 12
  ramps, railings, stairs,
    and grab bars, 12–13
  safety, 8–9
Hosiery, 32–34
Hospital discharge, 65
Hospital stays, 62–65
Hospital visitors, 64
Hotels, 83–86
Housecleaning, 18–19

Independent living centers,
    4–5
Internet, 3
Ironing, 19

Key devices, adaptive, 12
Kitchen appliances, 40

Kitchen working levels, 41
Knit fabrics, 35–36
Knives, 48

Labor-saving devices, 3–4
Large-Type Books in Print,
   72–73
Laundry, 19–20
Lever handles, 10
Light switches, 9–10
Lighting, 9–10
Lightweight dishes, 44
Locks and keys, 12
Low-fat diet, 44

Magnifying glass, 23
Making the bed, 16–17
Maternity clothes, 36–37
Meal planning and
   preparation, 42–44
Meals, air travel and, 79
Mealtime stress, 45
Mealtimes, 39–50
   adaptive devices, 48–50
   grocery shopping,
     46–48
   making the kitchen
     accessible, 40–42
   meal planning and
     preparation, 42–44
   serving meals, 44–46
Medical issues, 53–67
   doctors' appointments,
     54–58
   home health care, 65–67
   hospital stays, 62–65
   medications, and medical
     tests, 58–62
   record keeping, 53–54
   research, 53–54

Medical records, 53–54
Medical tests, 58–62
Medications, 58–62
Medicine chest mirror, 16
Medicine chest, organizing,
   15
Memory and concentration,
   improving, 67–72
Menu planning, 46
Motels, 83–86

Nail polish, 27
Napkins, 45
Necktie, tying, 29–30
Noise, coping with, 5
Nurse practitioner, as
   liaison, 57–58

Offset hinges, doorways,
   and 11
Oven-to-table cookware, 41

Packing, for travel, 82–83
Pantyhose, 28–29, 32
Passport, foreign travel and,
   82
Patient advocates, 64–65
Pegboards, for kitchen
   utensils, 41
Permanent press fabric, 35
Personal appearance, 25–38
   accessories, 37
   clothing alterations,
     30–32
   dressing tips, 28–30
   footwear, 32–34
   grooming, 26–27
   hosiery, 32–34
   shopping for clothes,
     34–37

Personal empowerment, 51–89
  medical issues, 53–67
  memory and concentration, 67–72
  restful activities, 72–75
  weekend getaways and extended travel, 75–89
Phone devices, 21–22
Photo cube, as telephone number holder, 23
Physician's assistant, as liaison, 57–58
Pill container, 61
Pizza, 45
Pocket organizer, 68
Power-dependent equipment, power outage and, 8
Prescription medications, travel and, 86–87
Prescription refills, 61

Railings, 12–13
Ramps, 12–13
Reachers, 3–4
Reading, 72–73
Reminder notes, 68
Remote controls, 74
Residence hotels and motels, 85–86
Resources, 91–102
  agencies and organizations, 94–97
  assistive technology, 97
  books, 93–94
  electronic information sources, 92–93
  environmental adaptations, 97–98
  information sources, 91–92
  speech impairment, 100–102
  travel, 98–99
  visual impairment, 100
Restful activities, 72–75
  games, 74–75
  reading, 72–73
  television, 73–74
Ricker-panel light switches, 9
Rugs, 18

Safety, 8–9
Scarf, cold weather and, 37
Scooters, 5
Seating chairs, 18
Serving meals, 44–46
Shoeboxes, 17–18
Shoemaker alterations, 33
Shopping by mail, 35
Shopping, clothes, 34–37
  choosing the right clothing, 35–37
  general tips, 34–35
Shopping, grocery, 5
Shoulder bag, 37
Shower adaptations, 14–15
Shower caddy, 14
Shower chairs, 15
Shower curtains, 10, 15
Shower nozzle, 15
Showering, 26
Sinks, 13–14
Sleeping positions, changing, 17
Slipper socks, 32
Slippers, 32
Snacks, travel and, 86

Stairs, 12–13
Stockings, 28–29
Storage cabinets, 41
Straws, drinking, 49
Suite hotels, 85
Support groups, 2–3
Support hose, 32
Sweeping, 18–19

Technology, time-saving, 3
Telephone cords, 22
Telephone, use of as
    intercom, 22
Television, 73–74
Thermal mugs, 48–49
Thermometer, 62
Three-wheeled scooter, air
    travel and, 80–81
Tissues, 16
Toenails, cutting, 27
Toilet seats, 14
Touch-sensitive lamps, 10
Travel resources, 87–89

Traveling, 75–89
    air travel, 79–82
    foreign travel, 82
    motels and hotels, 83–86
    packing, 82–83
    preparations, 75–77
    travel resources, 87–89
    traveling by car, 77–79
Traveling by car, 77–79
Traveling with children, 87
Tube socks, 32

Velcro, 31
Velcro-closing shoes, 33

Wall light switch extenders,
    9–10
Wash mitt, 16
Washcloths, 26
Water, taking medications
    and, 62
Weekend getaways, 75–87
Writing, 23

Demos Medical Publishing, Inc.
publishes numerous books on multiple sclerosis.
These include:

Multiple Sclerosis: A Guide for the Newly Diagnosed
Nancy J. Holland, T. Jock Murray, and Stephen C. Reingold

**Multiple Sclerosis: The Questions You Have—
The Answers You Need**
Rosalind C. Kalb

Multiple Sclerosis: A Guide for Families
Rosalind C. Kalb

Multiple Sclerosis: A Wellness Approach
George H. Kraft and Marci Catanzaro

Multiple Sclerosis: Your Legal Rights, 2nd ed.
Lanny E. Perkins and Sara Perkins

Employment Issues in Multiple Sclerosis
Phillip D. Rumrill, Jr.

Symptom Management in Multiple Sclerosis, 3rd ed.
Randall T. Schapiro

Therapeutic Claims in Multiple Sclerosis, 4th ed.
William A. Sibley

To receive additional information on these or any of our
other titles, call our toll-free number
(800) 532-8663

Demos Medical Publishing, Inc.
386 Park Avenue South
New York, New York 10016
Phone (212) 683-0072
Fax (212) 683-0118